MIMI KUO-DEEMER

XIU YANG

SELF-CULTIVATION FOR A HAPPIER, HEALTHIER AND BALANCED LIFE

First published in Great Britain in 2019 by Orion Spring
an imprint of The Orion Publishing Group Ltd
Carmelite House, 50 Victoria Embankment
London EC4Y 0DZ

An Hachette UK Company

1 3 5 7 9 10 8 6 4 2

Copyright © Mimi Kuo-Deemer, 2019
Illustrations by Emanuel Santos

The moral right of Mimi Kuo-Deemer to be identified as
the author of this work has been asserted in accordance
with the Copyright, Designs and Patents Act of 1988.

Diagram on page 48 © Jane Barthelemy www.fiveseasonsmedicine.com, used with
permission and thanks. Quotes on pages 26, 63–4, 91–2, 115, 137, 160, 186, 205 from
Handbooks for Daoist Practice: Inward Training (Hong Kong: Yuen Yuen Institute,
2008) © Louis Komjathy, used with permission and thanks. Quote on page 73 from
Original Tao, by Harold D. Roth. Copyright © 1999 Columbia University Press.
Reprinted with permission of Columbia University Press.
Image on page 78 courtesy of the Wellcome Collection.

Every effort has been made to ensure that the information in the book
is accurate. The information in this book may not be applicable in each
individual case so it is advised that professional medical advice is obtained
for specific health matters and before changing any medication or dosage.
Neither the publisher nor author accepts any legal responsibility for any
personal injury or other damage or loss arising from the use of the
information in this book. In addition, if you are concerned about
your diet or exercise regime and wish to change them, you
should consult a health practitioner first.

A CIP catalogue record for this book is
available from the British Library.

ISBN (Hardback) 978 1 4091 8397 6
ISBN (eBook) 978 1 4091 8398 3

Printed in Great Britain by Clays Ltd, Elcograf S.p.A.

To Aaron,

who brings laughter and love to my life.

Also in memory of Mayling,

who spread positivity and joy at every turn.

ABOUT TRANSLATIONS, LANGUAGE
AND TEXTS USED IN THIS BOOK

ON LANGUAGE: There are two types of English transliteration from Chinese: pinyin and Wade-Giles. In most cases, the worldwide standard of pinyin is used. Exceptions are when the Wade-Giles transliteration has fallen into common use in English, such as 'tai chi'. Traditional, or complex Chinese characters are also used instead of the simplified forms. When referencing Buddhist terminology, Pali is used and, when referencing yogic terminology, Sanskrit is used.

ON TEXTS USED: Many of the textual references used in *Xiu Yang* come from an ancient, early Daoist text known as *Inward Training (Neiye)*. This fourth-century BCE text is not well known, but is arguably the oldest mystical text in China. Though I also reference other more well-known Chinese classical texts such as the *Laozi*, or *Dao De Jing*, *Zhuangzi* and the *Confucian Analects* within this book, I have drawn particularly from *Inward Training (Neiye)* to illustrate the earliest sources and basis for self-cultivation in the Chinese tradition.* The mental and physical techniques for self-discipline in *Inward Training (Neiye)* were aimed at achieving physical health, longevity and spiritual transcendence. In other words, they sought to provide people a means to achieve a happier, healthier and more balanced way of living, which is also the goal of this book.

* Roth, 'Psychology and Self-Cultivation in Early Taoistic Thought', *Harvard Journal of Asiatic Studies* (1991), p. 611.

CONTENTS

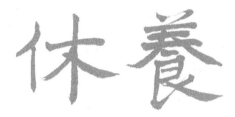

Xiu yang (pronounced 'sheow yaang') is the ancient Chinese art of self-cultivation. For centuries the aims of xiu yang have been improved health, a long and happy life, and harmony with the natural world. Xiu yang is the bedrock of Chinese healing and spiritual practices. The sages, emperors and spiritual seekers who have embraced xiu yang believed in smoothing out roughness and irregularities until our bodies and minds were nurtured, our energies strengthened, and our spirits integrated and guided by the forces of the natural world. At its core xiu yang asks us: what positive qualities do we wish to cultivate in our lives? It shows us that what we plant and grow can be the best in ourselves, which can also reflect overall goodness and well-being within society, nature and the universe. As an ancient wisdom xiu yang is a practice that we can follow today as a fundamental path towards a happier, healthier and balanced life.

FOREWORD

'A seed knows how to grow and flower,
humans have a similar capacity...'

A seed does indeed know how to grow and flower yet anyone
who has ever cultivated a garden also knows that nature best
rewards those who tend to their garden. Tending a garden is a
daily task: enriching the soil with manure, watering delicate
seedlings, watching for early signs of disease, protecting
plants from damaging winds and frosts, and harvesting fruits
and vegetables when they are at their peak ripeness. When
these tasks are done with careful attention and consistency,
it is wonderful to see how the garden glows with vitality and
rewards us with abundant and nutritious food. Yet after a few
weeks, months or years of neglect, that same garden has a way
of turning in the other direction: towards disarray, disease and
decay. Tending a garden is not much different from tending
one's home, tending a relationship or tending one's health.
If we regularly clean and tidy our home, it is a lovely and
calming place to live and to share with treasured guests. If we
invest time and energy in our relationships, we build enduring
connections that have a stronger chance of surviving the tests
of time. And nowhere are the results of consistent care more
obviously demonstrated than through the presence of good
health, mental clarity and joyfulness.

Yet today we face a worldwide health crisis of illnesses and diseases, which are largely the result of unbalanced lifestyle habits, poor diet and plain and simple lack of movement and exercise. We've been indoctrinated to believe that health and 'health insurance' are the purview of 'health practitioners', whose responsibility it is to treat our sicknesses and woes once they take hold. Within this cultural context, the simple yet profound message of xiu yang might easily be overshadowed, yet the urgency and relevance of this book will be apparent to anyone interested in cultivating and preserving their physical, mental and emotional well-being. The fundamental message of xiu yang is that to a large extent our health and happiness are within the domain of our own control, should we wish to exercise that sovereignty.

As a practice for 'smoothing out roughness and irregularity' and rekindling our innate wholeness and connection with nature, this offering of xiu yang, presented through a contemporary lens, could not have arrived at a better time. For who among us does not feel the tide-like pull of modern life's frantic pace from the moment we are awakened by our alarm clock to the moment we come to a skid stop in front of our bed and collapse into an often restless sleep? In between we may wrestle with the overwhelming information indigestion that occurs when we stuff ourselves from morning to night with input from our digital devices, while simultaneously juggling the immediate exigencies of our home, work and family responsibilities. But there is another way of living. This delightful book graciously offers us a view into what that might look like, and how, through simple, practical steps, we can reclaim harmony in our lives.

As I began reading *Xiu Yang*, I was immediately struck by the grounded kindness and the calm and measured pace of the voice of the author which, while invisible, is a palpable thread in between the lines of each word, each sentence and each beautifully crafted concept. Reading this book is, in itself, a therapeutic experience as one imbibes the direct experience of one who is living and breathing the message of xiu yang: self-cultivation for a happier, healthier and balanced life.

Throughout this exquisite book, Mimi Kuo-Deemer reminds the reader again and again to consider that self-cultivation is fundamentally different to self-care, which often translates as giving ourselves titbits of luxury such as a hot bath or a weekend getaway to remedy an otherwise self-abusing life. Self-cultivation on the other hand is a *way of life*. A painting we return to again and again to balance its colours, shapes and perspective. Self-cultivation is about finding a better balance within our self, with others and with the world.

The term xiu yang may at first appear to be a remote and foreign practice of little relevance to people outside of China. Yet it soon becomes clear that the fundamental concepts of xiu yang are readily applicable for anyone interested in building a sustainable life that is imbued with vibrant health, mental and emotional clarity, and the most basic human need of all: happiness.

Mimi gently guides the reader to attend to the breath, the body and the greater cultivation of qi, the animating life force that orchestrates harmony within the human body. Gradually she builds these foundation practices to include the deeper practices of mindfulness, as well as the more challenging practices of forgiveness and compassion. Throughout this text she uses the time-honoured tradition of storytelling to bring each of these concepts into the heart of the reader. Drawing from her own rich life experiences and those of her many students, the stories in this book move the heart and by doing so anchor understanding where it can best take root and thrive.

In writing this book Mimi is retrieving and archiving a treasure of wisdom that is at risk of being lost forever as China takes on many of the trappings of Western culture and jettisons its own historical healing modalities. Having bridged both cultures through living, working, studying and teaching in both Eastern and Western countries, Mimi has a unique ability to translate the subtle and sometimes elusive concepts of Chinese medicine, Confucian philosophy, Daoism, Buddhism and yoga into a coherent fabric. As Mimi says: 'Xiu yang is not about bandaging wounds or cleaning up after the damage is already done. It is about changing direction and going down a different path.' Know that, as you begin to read this book, you have a reliable guide to lead you in that new direction.

Donna Farhi

A Self that is Whole and Complete

For years I was an overworked, asthmatic, stressed-out photojournalist working in China. I travelled too much, smoked too much and was generally not great company. For starters, I was often sick. When my physical health began to take a serious turn for the worse, I realised that something had to change. At the beginning I assumed, like many people do, that to heal myself meant fixing myself and embarking on a path of self-improvement. What I have learned over time is that rather than seeing yourself as somehow damaged or flawed, you can remember that beneath the crusty layers of tension, tiredness or anxiety is an already intact sense of self that is whole and complete. One of my main yoga teachers, Donna Farhi, is one person who has helped me understand this. In her book, *Yoga Mind, Body and Spirit*, she tells us that yoga is a practice that deconstructs the barriers to experiencing our authentic self. In the book she writes: 'the effort to change and improve ourselves is fraught with the risk of subtle self-aggression that only produces more unhappiness. We cannot strive towards something that we already are.'[1]

Xiu yang's central aim is to help remind us not of our faults, but of our potential to experience a true sense of balance and well-being. When we feel this potential awaken, our lives are naturally enriched by deeper meaning and value. For myself, embracing the concepts of xiu yang has become a path to health that I never imagined possible fifteen years ago.

The beauty of xiu yang lies in its inherently simple and nature-based approach. Just as a fish knows how to hatch from its egg and start to swim, or a seed knows how to grow and flower, humans have a similar capacity to live well and feel lasting happiness and peace. We also have the capacity to feel spacious and vast, which is the opposite of feeling tight, contracted, small or separate. Yet because of the complex job of being a human being, our body, mind and heart can easily forget that they can be vast. Instead, they constrict and fragment daily, leaving us at times anxious, sad and confused.

The ancient Chinese were aware that our capacity to live freely was often compromised, which is why they aimed to rediscover a sense of balance, harmony and belonging in the world. They advised following certain approaches to exercise, diet and eating, sleep patterns, breathing, meditation and lovemaking. They also championed virtues such as kindness, generosity and compassion. Through adjusting these habits, we could begin to realign with the natural patterns and cycles of the universe. Nourishing and growing good habits and lifestyle choices was like preparing a field so that it would grow the healthiest, most sustainable crops.

The fundamental principles behind xiu yang tell us we cannot be in harmony with the world if we are not in harmony with ourselves. Regardless of age, state of health or circumstance, we all have an opportunity and ability to discover our inner balance, which manifests in outer radiance. These early ideas about xiu yang have translated across centuries and continue to influence the way many Chinese, especially those who follow traditions such as Confucianism, Daoism or Buddhism, approach their lives. It is also what I hope to offer in this book by exploring through a contemporary lens relevant and accessible practices you can do today.

A PRACTICE FOR THE HEART

Xiu yang is short for *xiu xin yang xin* (修心養心). In Chinese *xiu* means to cultivate, *yang* means to nurture, and *xin* means the heart. Xiu yang is therefore more than just self-cultivation; it is the practice of cultivating and nurturing one's heart. The heart is a rich and vast place. In many spiritual traditions, from Daoism to Buddhism and yoga, it represents infinite space, the seat of consciousness, the home of the eternal and the supreme sovereign. In Tibetan Buddhism the heart is home to a jewel. When the heart awakens, it radiates the light of compassion in all directions. When we undertake the cultivation and nurturing of our hearts, we have the potential to touch into its natural state of being open, clear, strong, compassionate and loving.

XIU YANG IN CHINA TODAY

Ask most Chinese people what xiu yang is, and they will say it is a quality rather than a process. Someone with xiu yang is a good, ethical and virtuous person. Growing up as the daughter of Chinese immigrant parents in the United States, this was what I also believed. While xiu yang can reflect one's character, for most of Chinese history it was understood as a process of cultivating a closer relationship with the natural world through spiritual and physical practices.

Most of these processes have been lost to people living in China today. This is partially because, until recently, mainland Chinese people saw Daoism and Confucianism – the systems from which xiu yang emerged – as weak ideological frameworks that led to the collapse of imperial Chinese rule. The impact of colonialism, modernisation and Communism over the last 150 years led many Chinese intellectuals as well as the general public to reject spiritual and religious practices as part of a feudal past that held China back from Western, scientific advancement. My parents were among those who saw meditation, qigong and other traditional approaches to cultivating one's self as backward and superstitious. In the last decade, however, this trend has begun reversing.[2] The number of new Daoist temples constructed has skyrocketed. Buddhist meditation and retreat centres are flourishing. People across mainland China are now beginning to reconnect the idea of xiu yang to its origins, which are to induce better physical health, a happier and more balanced heart, ethical clarity, and, at the highest levels, to achieve spiritual awakening. As this tide in the East begins to swell, my hope is it will help us in the West also begin to swim in these rich waters of wisdom.

SELF-CULTIVATION IN YOGA AND BUDDHISM

The Chinese were not alone in embracing the idea that we can cultivate positive qualities. Many Buddhist meditations and practices, such as developing compassion, kindness and joy, are known as *bhāvanā*, which means cultivation, development or 'bringing into being'. When we cultivate good qualities, they are believed to help us along the path towards greater insight, wisdom and awakening.

Yoga practitioners throughout the centuries have also embraced *bhāvanā* as a form of cultivating wholesome character traits. While historically there have been forms of yoga practice that veered towards drastic measures, such as self-starvation, holding the breath or raising one arm towards the sky for decades, there were also those who chose a gentler path. This was the path of *bhāvanā*. As we explore xiu yang, we will also be considering some of these softer approaches from yoga and Buddhism as ways to introduce resources for better living.

AN ANCIENT, INCLUSIVE TRADITION

Who can practise xiu yang? Anyone. Throughout Chinese history Daoist priests, Buddhist nuns, Confucian scholars and government officials were all on the xiu yang bandwagon. How was this possible? Unlike the contentious history between Christianity and Islam, the Chinese religious tradition has allowed many beliefs to co-exist peacefully for centuries. Though less true in mainland China today, if you go to London's or New York City's Chinatown, Hong Kong or Malaysia, a typical temple scene involves people bowing to a statue of Confucius, praying to Tian Hou, the Daoist Queen of Heaven, and giving a final offering to the Buddhist Guanyin, or Bodhisattva of Compassion.

For most of Chinese history rarely has one tradition had to prove itself better than another. This is an especially important example to remember in today's world, where strong identification and attachment to certain traditions or lineages of practice can often end up separating and pitting spiritual practitioners against each other. What this means is that xiu yang is a practice open to everyone. You do not have to have any specific background or affiliation to embrace xiu yang; you only need to remember that you are part of the natural world and have the potential to grow what is of deeper meaning and value in your life.

HARMONY IN THE WORLD THROUGH HARMONY WITHIN OURSELVES

Xiu Yang is organised into four parts:

Part 1: The Art of Xiu Yang;

Part 2: Xiu Yang for a Healthy and Harmonious Body;

Part 3: Xiu Yang for a Balanced Mental and Emotional Life;

Part 4: Xiu Yang for a Happier Place in the World.

Part 1 will guide you through an understanding of the Dao and its relationship to xiu yang's aims. It will also present the mandala of xiu yang. A mandala is a ritual symbol representing the universe. It is typically drawn with circles inside squares. The mandala of xiu yang will provide a map of inner balance, leading to outward peace in your life. This map will help you sharpen your senses and see the ways you can practise self-cultivation in any moment. It will also help you orientate your practices as you move through the book.

In Part 2, xiu yang for the body, we will explore how to align with the natural rhythms of the day and explain the importance of moderate exercise, healthy breathing and the role of diet from a xiu yang perspective. Part 3 looks at getting to know your heart and mind more fully through the Buddha's teachings on mindfulness. In better understanding your heart you can begin to appreciate and love those in your life and community with greater care and compassion, which is the focus of Part 4.

As you read through this book, some of the ideas may be inspiring or immediately valuable. Others may seem beyond reach. Think of the immediately inspiring ideas or ways to begin cultivating aspects of yourself as flowers you can buy from the nursery and bring home to place at your windowsill and see daily. For the sections that you may read and think, 'Now that is a good idea, but not realistic for me to think about right now', put them into the category of seeds or bulbs that you can keep in the greenhouse and one day grow.

Importantly, as you read through this book, please do not take my or anyone else's words as absolute truth. Rather, do as the Buddha advised: *Ehipassiko* – or 'Come and see for yourself'.[3] Investigate, inquire and explore these teachings in the light of your own reasoning, practice and insight. This will be the best confirmation of whether these practices hold value, potency and meaning for you.

FROM SELF-CARE
TO SELF-CULTIVATION

When we begin to work with xiu yang, it's important to consider that self-cultivation is different from self-care. Self-care can sometimes be seen as a short-term solution to our difficulties: after a hard day we soak in a hot bubble bath or treat ourselves to something like a massage, watching a romcom or having some ice cream. While self-care is essential, we can also begin to see that we need deeper, lasting solutions to supporting our long-term health and well-being.

Xiu yang is not about bandaging wounds or cleaning up after the damage is already done. It is about changing direction and going down a different path. It is looking at what it means to be human in this world, with the different roles and responsibilities you undertake. It is asking: how do I make my way through this world as naturally, clearly and awake as I can be? It is going back to the source of yourself and seeing what aspects of your heart you can cultivate and nurture to help reach the depth and radiance of your inner being. Xiu yang helps you see where self-cultivation can lead you: an embrace of a sense of self that is not fragmented, separate and damaged, but part of the totality of this universe that is always whole and complete.

PART 1

The Art of Xiu Yang

I often think of the source underlying the beauty of the natural world. How did the variety, balance and colours of a sunset, wildflower or autumn leaf become such high art? When looking at nature and her exquisite designs, I am often struck by an 'articulate speechlessness', or an experience that transcends my attempt to interpret what is happening.[4] Some call this source by a name, such as science, God or love. For the ancient Chinese sages the source of the natural world was understood as the Dao.

To them the Dao could only be known through cultivating moment-to-moment experience. Like the unending canvas of the sky opening to the stars, they saw the great creation of our lives as infinite and full of possibility. Xiu yang is the means through which you can know this possibility. It orientates your aspirations to connect to what is around you as fully and authentically as you can. As you do this, you discover ways to soften your resistance to the challenges of life while aligning with the potential of who you can become. This is the art of xiu yang.

1

Xiu Yang and the Dao

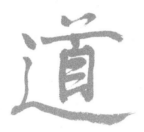

Xiu yang brings the Dao to life for human beings. It allows us to feel at one with the Dao and its evolving, living impulses. Just as a seed requires nourished soil, water and sunlight to grow into a sprout and mature into a flowering plant, our bodies, minds and spirits require certain beneficial conditions to mature and grow with less friction and more ease. With xiu yang you begin to identify ways you can live more in tune with the Dao's natural unfolding.

What is the Dao? Most simply, it is the power that underlies all continuing patterns of the universe. Naturalness, effortlessness and simplicity lie at the heart of the Dao. It is believed to unfold shapelessly and fluidly. In the *Dao De Jing* (also known as *Tao Te Ching*), a widely translated book outlining the central themes of Daoism, it is a nameless force that is hard to define yet which gives rise to all things.

The Dao is often equated to water: it is endlessly self-replenishing, soft yet deeply powerful. At its essence it is good and fundamentally benevolent. The Dao is defined as great and present at the beginning of heaven and earth. It is also humble: it flows to the lowest places and nourishes all things without ever being asked. It gives life to all but asks for nothing in return, benefits everything without taking sides, rules yet asserts no authority.[5] It moves in cyclical, spherical forms, which contrasts to today's linear, goal-orientated tendencies of humans. Some describe the Dao as an intangible energy that moves and resides everywhere yet can also suddenly be at rest; in these moments it resides in the heart.[6]

NOTHING IS SEPARATE

The guiding principle of the Dao is that all experience is relative; nothing exists in complete isolation or separation. One thing exists only in relationship to something else. This means that nothing in itself is long or short; if we define one thing as long, it is only longer than something else we take as a standard. The same is true of inner and outer, beautiful or ugly, thrilling or dull. As the *Dao De Jing* describes:

> *Being and non-being create each other;*
> *Difficult and easy complete each other;*
> *Long and short contrast one another;*
> *High and low rest upon each other;*
> *Tones and sounds blend with each other;*
> *Before and after follow one another.*[7]

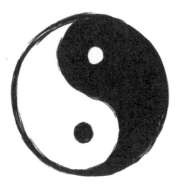

The yin/yang symbol best illustrates these ideas of relativity, balance and wholeness. It shows how opposites co-exist within the totality that is the Dao. Yin is shade, receptivity, contraction, density and darkness. Yang is brightness, activity, expansion, refinement and light. These opposing forces work to create harmony and continuity.

The characters for yin and yang were originally defined as the shady and sunny side of a mountain. Ancient Daoist and shamanic sages observed that as the sun rose and crossed the sky, one side of the mountain would be lit by sun as the other side remained in shadow. By afternoon the pattern would reverse as the sun continued its journey towards darkness, leaving the morning's sunny side in shade and its shaded side in sun. Through the interplay of yin and yang a natural harmony in the world as well as in our lives can be discovered.

How does this perspective relate to xiu yang? Each time you meet a tricky situation, such as feeling slighted, judged or otherwise uncomfortable, you also remember *that nothing is separate.* The Dao teaches that all contrasts are harmonised and opposites blended together to become a whole. This helps you begin to see that while you may think your opinions are different to others', or others are wrong and you are right, this is not the truth. With the Dao you are invited to see context. You remember that you are not isolated from others but part of a living, breathing matrix that defines and shapes all living beings. Completeness and unity are always present. They constitute our most fundamental nature, and are always accessible. Xiu yang helps you recognise this.

This model for unity, importantly, helps you maintain perspective through life. Implicit within the darkness of yin is the light of yang. Within the lightness of yang the dark of yin is accepted and understood. This can help you bear in mind that when you are struggling in life, no matter how great the pain, you can still let in light. Likewise, if you are thriving and happy in life, you remember not to turn away from or exclude the possibility of discomfort or loss. Xiu yang gives you the mental and physical discipline necessary to help keep this vantage point. It lets you recognise that your experience is not fragmented or divided, but a dance of opposites. Some days you will be in sun, and other days in shade. This does not change the totality of your being.

Deeper understandings of the relationship between yin and yang are at the core of many spiritual teachings. It helps us see that sadness and happiness can arise simultaneously, as can joy and pain. We also understand that with life there is death. Nothing can exist without the other. When we accept this approach to experience, we can begin to let go of hoping for pleasure and struggling against pain.

In 2015 there were a series of terrorist attacks in Paris and then Berlin. The tragedies reminded me of a powerful teaching from the classic yogic text, the *Yoga Sūtra*: *pratipaksha bhavanam*.[8] It means cultivating the opposite perspective, especially when there are strong, difficult emotions present. A student had asked me about this idea in the wake of the attacks, and this is what I wrote to her in response:

> *Pratipaksha bhavanam* helps keep perspective that events operate on a spectrum. Sometimes the pendulum can swing to one extreme end of emotions, and we forget that while we feel despair there is also happiness and beauty. In a talk I heard by Richard Freeman he spoke about *pratipaksha bhavanam* as exemplified beautifully in vinyasa – the movement of upward dog is followed by downward dog, the in breath is always followed by the out breath. Thank goodness we are never stuck in upward-facing dog forever! We have the perspective and experience of its complement and opposite. In Sri Swami Satchidananda's translation of the *Sūtra* he also describes inviting opposite thoughts to help defuse negative thinking patterns.[9] When we feel hatred or anger, we think about love or look at a beautiful image.
>
> When tragedy like a terrorist attack takes place, it is not that we turn away from the grief, sadness, fear or anger. It is that we remember that for all the tragedy happening there is also beauty. I have been

quite moved these past few days by the posts and stories of how communities have come together to give blood, offer shelter, check in on loved ones, and work towards being more kind every day. The outpouring of love, hope and faith is encouraging and brave. This is a beautiful practice of *pratipaksha bhavanam*. May this help us keep perspective and context, and encourage our ability as human beings to grow and change.

Can life be beautiful? Yes, it can be heaven on earth. Can life be horrible? Yes. It can be like a hellhole. Both of these are true, and the two co-exist. Side by side, yin and yang give you the ability to break free from a one-sided view of life. When you only choose to see life and not death, or only hope for heaven on earth but not hell, then imbalance and suffering arise. Balance is seeing both possibilities as valid and part of the whole.

XIU YANG FOR EXPERIENCING BALANCED WHOLENESS

This is a simple exercise to help you work with the idea of wholeness. Take a moment in your day to look at a shadow from a tree, person or building. When you see the shadow, you only see it because there is sunlight. Then shift your attention to light. Try to absorb yourself in the light. Is it possible? Can you only see the light without the shadow? Chances are from your perspective it is impossible to only see one and not the other. When you next face a difficult situation, use this example to try to see your situations in the same way: if you are sad, look at the beauty of a flower or the sky. If you are frustrated, consider what is fluid and free, like your ability to breathe or see wind blowing in trees. Let these contrasts slowly harmonise your experience so that all combines into a blended whole.

HOLDING THE VIEW OF VASTNESS

You may think this is strange or completely normal, but I regularly ask trees for advice. Often, I choose old, tall trees that have been around for a while – hundreds, perhaps even thousands of years. On one occasion, while hiking in the Swiss Alps, I saw an enormous pine at the top of a ridge. Without hesitation I knew this tree would grant me valuable insights or wisdom. Respectfully, I approached the tree, rested my head against its wide, scaled trunk, and presented my question: 'Is there anything I need to know?' Immediately, I heard an ancient voice echo these words: 'Stay vast.'

I have taken this advice to heart. Every day, whenever I can remember, I aspire to let vastness shape my outlook. Vastness is the opposite of feeling tight, contracted, small or separate. Yet because of the complicated, messy job of being human, our body, mind and heart can easily forget that they can be vast. Instead, they constrict and fragment daily, leaving us at times anxious, sad and confused.

Vastness is a feeling you might have a glimpse of when fully absorbed in a profound event: a birth, a death, a marriage or a sunrise. In these moments time stands still, and your mind quietens. In moments where you see beyond your thoughts and into deeper meaning, you can feel inclusive and spacious. Truth is no longer camouflaged. Instead, you feel something honest. You feel *yourself*. You may even sense that you are part of something greater than you could ever imagine.

Unfortunately, we often think of these moments as seren-dipitous. As pure chance, they arise and pass. What if you considered, however, that these moments of clear perception are not just chance? What if this recognition of vastness was intrinsic? What if feeling happy, whole and like we belong to a larger life were possible in more moments throughout your day?

Holding the view of vastness helps you recognise that you always have a choice when confronting your personal dramas. It is also a hallmark of xiu yang: through a steady cultivation of your awareness, you can make a mental shift from whatever causes you to feel small, separated and isolated, and open to a vast and limitless view of life. This can feel like a surge of freedom.

XIU YANG FOR THE VIEW OF VASTNESS: SHIFT FROM SMALL SELF TO A LARGER LIFE

Be on the listen for when your mind is caught up in small, petty concerns. Often this happens when we are with people we don't know well, but it can also happen with colleagues and family. The Buddha called this the 'I me mine' tendency of thought that traps us into selfish desires of clinging to how things should be, or pushing away things we do not like. When we are caught up in stories about ourselves, we become myopic, contract inwards, and lose touch with the larger view of life. We can become so consumed by our problems that we forget that we are not the most important thing in the world. The Beatles sang about the Buddha's teachings in a song called 'I Me Mine', which debuted on their album *Let It Be*. The song lyrics tell us that 'Ev'ryone's saying it … I me mine,' and describe how widespread our tendency to be caught up in small concerns is.

If you notice being caught up in a sense of small self, try making a mental shift to something spacious: the openness of sky, sunlight through a window or the mystery that each person is breathing, conscious and part of creation. Or perhaps conjure the echoes of a giant pine's advice to stay vast. In this way you can begin to move from a sense of small self to a larger life.

THE SPIRIT HORSE AND *WU WEI*

The lynchpin of Daoist thought is a Chinese concept known as *wu wei* (無為). *Wu wei* means effortless action. It does not mean being passive or disinterested, but rather determining how much force is necessary to accomplish a task. It means effort without struggle, actions that avoid unnecessary thrashing

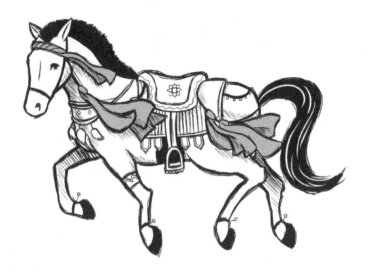

around, not wasting energy to accomplish what you need to do in life. Think of a tightrope walker who requires complete and relaxed focus to remain balanced, or a martial artist who stays calm and alert in the midst of a fight. *Wu wei* arises when we are in the flow of experience. It is the antithesis to strife and struggle.

One of my favourite stories of *wu wei* in action happened while I was working as a photographer in 2004. I was assigned to a project in the remote regions of eastern Tibet. One day, I took a drive with some colleagues towards the even more remote regions of the province near the Bhutanese border. Halfway there our car, a sturdy but aged Land Rover, broke down. Initially, we weren't concerned; all Land Rovers come with a spare tyre on the back in case of situations such as this.

As our driver tried to loosen the bolt holding the tyre in place, however, he began to struggle. The bolt was rusted and would not budge. Others in the car took turns trying to free the screw. We flagged down a rare passing car stuffed with Chinese officials; some of them wore armed police uniforms. Each of the strong men wrestled to free the tyre, but none succeeded. Their efforts began to strip the bolt, and hope of freeing the tyre began to wane. The late-afternoon light started to fade.

Everyone was exhausted. None of us were prepared for the dropping temperatures or impending darkness. Between the four of us we only had a bit of water and some trail mix I had taken as a last-minute snack. Eventually a car drove by with a free seat and offered to take one of our colleagues back to town. We had no idea when he would be back. Nightfall was only an hour or so away.

Meanwhile, two young Tibetan nomads had seen us from a distance. They wore plastic sandals with yak wool-lined coats. After some time their curiosity lured them closer. They sat at a distance, watching all the large, strong men use their body weight and force to try to wrench the bolt free. When they saw them give up, they moved in closer. One of the Tibetans, who looked no older than seventeen, offered to try. Most of us had given up hope of freeing the tyre by then, and few paid him much attention. After all, if the armed police could not free the tyre, who could?

The nomad set to work quietly. My curiosity was piqued, so I went to see what he was doing. He had carefully placed the wrench on the bolt. He positioned the wrench in such a way that would prevent further stripping. He would shift his weight to effect different leverage, and wait for tiny responses. His persistence and listening attention paid off. Slowly the bolt began to turn. Within another five minutes he had freed the screw.

As he was working, a beautiful white horse decorated with bells and ribbons arrived. By this point we were all watching the nomad, but the delicate hoofs and singing bells that announced the horse's arrival drew my attention. The driver was an older cheerful and rosy-cheeked Tibetan who stopped to watch.

I sometimes think about this horse as a spirit horse. I sensed that his calm, majestic presence offered unspoken support to the young nomad as he worked the bolt loose. I remember how he responded to the resistance that had trapped the bolt. Rather than forcing and demanding that the bolt be free of the years of rust and resilience that had accumulated, he quietly felt for the right amount of effort necessary to work it free. He embraced softness and abandoned the need for might. He showed no conflict or struggle, but instead was at ease and relaxed. He had practised the art of *wu wei*. This was xiu yang in action.

Ancient Indian texts often use the horse as a way to understand our mind.[10] The horse is described as our senses. Senses directly impact our thoughts. If our senses are left running free, they become unpredictable and wild like an untrained horse that never obeys its rider. When the senses, however, are quiet and trained, the horse moves through its path with less fear. In time it learns to respond calmly and steadily to its rider and makes peace with its environment. The willingness to train and quieten the senses is also xiu yang.

This story is a reminder that too much effort or force is not always useful, especially when meeting a mind that is restless and confused, or a body that is resistant to a complex shape. But just like the armed police who tried to push, strain and force the bolt of the tyre free, our natural tendency in meeting something that simply will not budge is often to overexert our efforts and then give up. If we can meet barriers with the presence of a calm spirit, however, we may find space to soften, listen and respond with the right amount of strength. In time we may also begin to train our attention to see whatever situation we face – during practice or everyday life – with less unnecessary force and more capacity for tuning in. We begin to discover we can cultivate this attitude and approach to life in any moment, enabling us to see what is arising in us and how we can respond most appropriately.

With xiu yang and the principle of *wu wei* given to us by the Dao we can foster resources that help us loosen the bolts and screws that tighten our bodies and mind without stripping them. We can work towards a balance of seeing our experiences more clearly so that we can be, breathe and live our lives more freely.

XIU YANG FOR *WU WEI*: NOT STRIPPING THE SCREW

The next time you do any exercise, whether that be going to the gym, doing a run or practising yoga or qigong, what would it feel like to use enough effort to affect your body without metaphorically stripping your screw? The same idea can be applied in meditation: sit with what is arising in your experience, and notice whether you can pay attention to your breathing, thoughts and sensations without trying to push them away or tighten around them more. Instead, let them be, responding to them with gentleness and listening.

The Buddha called this approach 'right effort' (*sammā vāyāma*). This means what you do is not too tight, and not too loose. From the teachings of the Dao this is *wu wei*: effortless action. Yoga defines this as the important pairing of doing your practice (*vairaghyam*) and stepping back from the outcome (*abhyasa*).

2

The Mandala of Xiu Yang

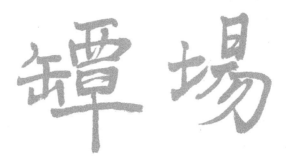

Mandalas are maps, and when learning to practise the art of xiu yang it can be helpful to have a lie of the land. They are ritual symbols used to establish meditative awareness, concentration and transcendence in many traditions, including yoga, Buddhism and Daoism. Mandala means 'circle'. Created using repeating geometric shapes of circles and squares within

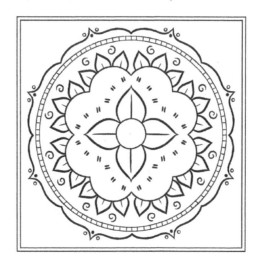

each other, mandalas typically represent a microcosm of the macrocosm: the square is nature or the universe, the circles are your experiences, and the centre is yourself. With these general orientations people can look at mandalas and know where they are in the universe.

THE MANDALA OF XIU YANG: BODY, HEART, MIND, WORLD

The symbolism of the mandala can help you see your place in the sacred space of everyday life. As a microcosm of the macrocosm, you are not just your mind and body but part of everything that moves, lives and breathes. You can begin to see connections and relationships to all that is around you. You don't just eat: by eating mindfully you remind yourself that what you consume was grown by the sun, rain and soil. You don't just exercise, but understand that movement can become a prayer to the temple of your body, navigating the gravitational pull between the earth and sky. You do not just speak, but consider how your speech ripples into the hearts and minds of others.

When considering the mandala as a model, I began to think about mapping what matters most in my life. To me, priorities are lasting happiness, health and balance. Yet how can I cultivate and grow these qualities? What are the sources for these? Family, friends and community initially come to mind as sources, as do health and well-being. But as much as we love family we can also feel excruciatingly hurt and betrayed by them. Friends and community often change, and our health is frequently challenged by demands from responsibilities and work. What, then, fits into the mandala of xiu yang that can lead to a lasting happiness?

The answer is that the true sources of happiness are within you and are capable of being grown. This is counter to the media messages we hear – that the latest phone, a piece of cake or a beach holiday will give us joy, satisfaction and comfort.

Unfortunately, external resources are short-lived; while nice to have and potentially assuaging of initial discomfort, invariably they fall short of becoming a reliable genesis of lasting happiness.

We will take a closer look at what lasting happiness is in Part 4, but in looking at the mandala of xiu yang, you can start by considering that the goals of self-cultivation help you tap into an internal spring of wisdom, compassion, steadfastness and generosity that is always available in ample supply as the Dao. This source of happiness enables you to meet the external world with clarity and lasting joy.

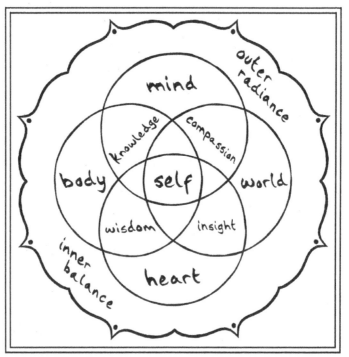

mandala of xiu yang — self-cultivation

READING YOUR MANDALA

In looking at your mandala of xiu yang, start with the notion that everything is related and part of the Dao. In this way your body's health will affect your mind and heart; how you act in the world will affect your body; what you think will impact your heart; and how you breathe will affect your thoughts.

Knowing this, start to navigate the map of your mandala in this way:

1. See the square as representative of the natural world and the Dao.

2. See yourself as part of this existence that is whole and complete.

3. Consider each aspect of yourself – body, mind, heart and world – and how they affect your self and vice versa.

4. Consider how ideas such as knowledge, wisdom, insight and compassion are products of how you meet your body, mind, heart and world, and vice versa.

5. Consider that your inner balance can lead to outer radiance, and outer radiance comes from inner balance.

6. See everything arising within yourself that is also part of the world around you.

CIRCLES AND SQUARES

If people are able to be aligned and still,
Their skin will be ample and smooth,
Their ears and eyes will be acute and bright
Their sinews will be supple, and their bones will be strong.
Then they will be able to hold up the Great Circle,
And they will tread firmly on the Great Square.

Inward Training (Neiye), Chapter 16[11]

The mandala of xiu yang places you in the centre, surrounded by a circle that represents your deeper self, which is always whole and complete.[12] Within the circle are four qualities that transform your inner self but also extend outwards to the world. These are knowledge, compassion, wisdom and insight. The outer square represents nature as whole and complete. In this model you interface with nature through your body, mind, heart and interactions, or your worldly relationships. As you aspire to guide and grow yourself into realising your potential as part of nature, you can begin to awaken your ability to be more fully human. Seeing yourself as part of these facets can be a powerful visual aid.

Body

Your body's health feeds yourself, but also your mind, heart and relationship to the world. Though initially you may focus on your body to change it – for example, you want it to be lighter, healthier or less tense – with xiu yang we will approach the body as a whole, and understand that it is affected by how we organise our day, when we eat or sleep, and how we choose activities depending on seasons and life cycles. Rather than seeing the body as something that needs fixing, we will explore the body as a seed that, given the right conditions, can grow and thrive. This exploration will be our journey for Part 2 of this book: 'Xiu Yang for a Healthy and Harmonious Body'.

Mind and heart

The mind is a wonderful thing: it allows you to reason, think, imagine, create and logically analyse experience. Thoughts are valuable and necessary. Yet much of the time what you think can be harmful and undermine you. When you begin to observe your thoughts, you start to discern what your thoughts actually are as they arise, and with this you create a wiser relationship with your mind. Are your thoughts judgemental or kind? Logical or random? Lost in the past or caught up with future concerns? With Part 3 of this book, 'Xiu Yang for a Balanced Mental and Emotional Life', we will look at how to grow the seeds of your good thoughts, and weed out those that wound and damage you.

We will also look at how to meet, open and expand your heart, which is often seen in Chinese philosophy, yoga and Buddhism as the same as the mind. The difference, however, between your *thinking life* and what your heart feels and metabolises *as life* merits closer attention. When you begin to cultivate your heart, you invite it to become what it is believed to do naturally when in balance: be open, wise and compassionate. This helps you weather emotional storms that often sweep across your internal landscape, and meet them with greater resource, courage and grace.

World

Human beings are relational creatures that are often burdened by tension, heartache, anger or fear. How can you cultivate a happier place in the world, especially with issues such as environmental devastation, extreme political views and mounting ethnic, racial and religious conflict? You can begin by considering that, as much as the world may feel in a shambles, it is also where you can go to find solutions. Throughout Chinese history xiu yang has fostered the idea that living in the world can be ethical, fluid, humble and spacious. The Buddha knew the importance of ethics, and prioritised it in his teachings. In fact, an ethical way of being in the world is the first stage of awakening. When you approach living with others ethically, you can also see that community becomes a source of great strength.

Understanding the interdependence of how these roles affect who you are is the key to xiu yang's unique approach to living: *you are not a linear development but rather a process of widening circles and squares, where everything is related to the centre.* You do not simply change your diet to improve your health. Rather, you improve your health through body, mind and spirit, which can shape your diet. You can also see that your diet affects what you practise and how you meet adversity. In other words, diet will move out as ripples on the surface of water, affecting and perhaps even determining the ways your body, mind, heart and role in the world unfold. These four areas directly affect the self but also grow out of the self; each is a part of the whole.

Cultivating clear ethics is rarely easy, but it is all the harder to do if our hearts and minds are confused, or our body depleted and unwell. Likewise, our hearts and minds may not be nourished without clear ethics, and we may not see the value of caring for our body without embracing an attitude of kindness, spaciousness and fluidity towards ourselves and the world.

THE LONG-TERM SUPPORT FOR OUR HAPPINESS

As you undertake the practices of self-cultivation, you also nourish four qualities that transform you at deeper levels. These are knowledge, compassion, wisdom and insight. The immediate differences between these qualities, particularly between knowledge, wisdom and insight, are not always clear. In fact, these four have distinct relationships with each other that I believe support true happiness. Through my personal reflection on these ideas I believe each has an effect and correlation on the other.

Knowledge

Learning facts and information from reading, listening and experiencing is part of a good education. Whether you are aware of it or not, you are always acquiring information that grows into knowledge. This is useful as it helps you gain context and make choices. Knowledge gives you the chance to gain new skills in life, and have a practical as well as theoretical understanding of what you do in a job or situation. Knowing, for example, who to call and what to do when your car breaks down is helpful knowledge to keep. For xiu yang we need knowledge to help us navigate our choices and deepen skills that help us grow.

Compassion

It is easy in life to become self-critical or compare oneself to others. This is why compassion is of vital importance when you work with the gradual process of self-cultivation. With compassion you see that any tendencies to be harsh, angry, confused or feel like you are falling short are not fundamental parts of who you are. Learning to meet these tendencies compassionately will soften and dissolve harshness. When you cultivate compassion, you begin to see that the things that poison your mind or heart are just visitors, rather than permanent residents. In the words of compassion expert Sharon Salzberg, these poisons are 'adventitious, not inherent'.[13] They are like pests or weeds that encroach on our fields. Compassion protects your garden from harm.

Wisdom

Wisdom is the quality that helps people communicate with care, sensibility and understanding. Knowledge is accumulated information, but wisdom is what applies our knowledge in ways that avoid being reckless or rash. It is having soundness of judgement. It arises out of contemplation of and reflection on all that you know. Wisdom is also what tells you there is still much to know.

Insight

When you gain the necessary knowledge and begin to use it wisely and compassionately, you open to insight. Insight is the ability to see into a situation with deeper understanding that comes through wisdom and knowledge. Insight is personal, and often the result of understanding the inner nature of things. It is introspection. Some consider insights truths; the Buddha's awakening, for example, is described as his insight into the true nature of experience. Part of this insight was to understand that all things change; yet another equally important insight is that while suffering exists and there is reason for it, there is also a path that leads us away from it and results in its end. This fundamental truth is what xiu yang can teach you to help you live.

LOVE MOVES AS THE PULSATION OF THE DAO

Through the mandala of xiu yang, we can see how different sections on the map also reflect a wider circle of experience. Just as Chinese people since ancient times have believed that the Dao is inherently benevolent, the Buddha taught that our minds and hearts are naturally radiant and pure. When you visualise yourself at the centre of the mandala, you can see what you cultivate is inner balance. This not only becomes a source of strength, centredness and grounding, but also a source of love.

From the perspective of Chinese philosophy love moves as the pulsation of the Dao. This pulsation is not passionate or sentimental, but an unobstructed source of energy that connects you to a part of yourself that is whole and complete. It is sunlight on water, wind heard in trees or a child's laughter. It is the mysterious power that creates, transforms and returns. It is the sublime feeling of seeing nature in its full, resplendent glory. Another way to see love is how the Buddha defined love, which is what he called *mettā*: the quality of a limitless heart that wishes no enmity or hate, but rather that all who live have a happy heart.[14] He believed that our ability to love springs from our true nature.

I witnessed the potential of this love arise within myself when facing the reality and pain of my sister-in-law's terminal cancer. For years we had a difficult relationship that was complicated by my father's death, her sickness and an inability to see past our mutual blame of each other for the pain we felt. This came to a head after a number of misunderstandings led to a screaming phone call where we nearly cut our relationship off completely. During a long silence where I was certain she would say, 'I never want to speak to you again', I summoned all my hours of meditation, yoga and qigong, and thought deeply about what was at the root of my anger and pain. Though my heart was teetering, and I felt my inner balance shaken, I managed to ask myself, 'What really matters right now, and why do I care so much?' Immediately, the answer was: 'She is family. I am hurt because I want her to love me, and I want to love her.' Rallying my reserves of courage and strength, I said, 'Rachael, it breaks my heart that you feel that I have not been compassionate or caring towards you. It was never my intention. I am sorry if I made you feel this way. I was so happy when you married John and I finally had a sister. I would like to understand what happened to us to make us so hurt, angry and confused.' In an instant she softened. We began to speak from our hearts. In the end we each promised to try to repair our relationship. Before she died I flew out to be with her and my brother's family. Though she was already unconscious, I felt a peace in my heart telling her that I loved her and that we found a way to appreciate each other again. I will always be grateful for her fierce willingness to open her heart and extend her love.

With the art of xiu yang we begin to reclaim our true potential: a natural way of being, breathing, living, loving and returning. With this we have the ability to reintroduce inner balance and true joy to life that is inherently ours to claim. When this begins to manifest, it effortlessly ripples out as health, happiness and outer radiance.

MANDALA VISUALISATION EXERCISE

Take a moment to look at the mandala of xiu yang on page 24. What is the square that is the natural world like for you? Are you connected to nature, or do you feel separate from it? How do the experiences of your body, mind, heart and relationships exist within the natural world right now? Imagine that each of these four aspects of yourself is in harmony with the ever-present feeling of the Dao, which is always whole and complete. Then take your attention to the circle, which is a representation of your complete and unfractured self. How do concepts such as knowledge, compassion, wisdom and insight sit with your sense of self? How do these play out in your body, mind, heart and world? Envision yourself as seated in the centre with these qualities rippling towards yourself at the centre, and then the rippling of these qualities from yourself back outwards. Continue imagining all these factors around you and within you, ebbing and flowing like the tides.

3

Seeing the Ordinary as Extraordinary

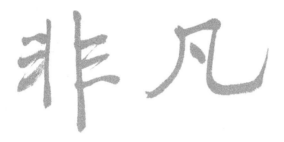

When we buy vegetables from a market or eat a salad from a store, we rarely consider it grew from a tiny seed nestled deep in rich soil. I certainly have consumed many a meal quickly and with little regard for the process that grew my food. Recently, however, my husband and I have begun to grow much of our own food. Knowing that the simple act of planting a seed into soil can produce a full, healthy head of lettuce gives me new insight into the process that leads to enjoying a mouthful of crispy freshness. Doing this has reminded me of how easily we can overlook the process of self-cultivation: when we feel genuinely healthy or happy, we can miss the simple, ordinary steps and stages that led to us becoming that way.

For much of its history China has been a farming society. Respect for the land has shaped and defined much of Chinese thinking. When I first visited China in 1984, I remember seeing rice paddies ploughed by farmers riding ox-driven carts. Many of these rice fields created stunning terraces that carved, shaped and informed the terrain; they flowed along the slopes of mountains like concentric ripples of water. This system of farming was an ancient example of a fully integrated ecosystem where plants, animals and humans created mutually sustainable resources for living. Very likely the farmers of these fields had tilled and tended to their land in this way for centuries.

Though much has changed in modern times, and today over half of China's population live in urban centres, ancient farming techniques still exist in regions of south-west China. These techniques have enabled water to be conserved, while supporting the lives of a number of aquatic animals and plants. Farmers prioritise perennial crops that prevent weeds from growing while protecting and nourishing the soil. Many contemporary trends in farming today, such as permaculture, look to achieve a similar interrelationship of organisms and their environments as Chinese people did with traditional gardening techniques. While most Chinese farmers have left this integrated approach behind, a number of agricultural communities continue to work with methods and tools that feed and nourish the land without disturbing its balance with pesticides or large machinery. Xiu yang shows that you too can create balance by cultivating your internal field naturally and holistically.

TAN CHANG: THE FIELD OF AN ALTAR

In China the mandala represents what is known as the 'field of an altar', or *tan chang* (壇場). An altar is a sacred place where people give offerings, pray and connect to spirit. It is a place for rituals. A field is an area of open land or pasture where humans walk, crops are planted and animals graze. Joining these ideas together – as the ancient Chinese sages did – forges the sacred with the natural, the spiritual with the everyday.

When most people look at an empty field of dirt, however, they may see little more than dried earth. In our language dirt has negative connotations, often meaning rotten, muddy or

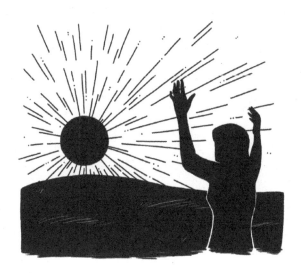

impure. Think of getting the dirt on someone's past, dirty movies or dirty laundry. Yet soil is something different. It is not impure. It is mysterious and life-giving. Its decomposed matter gives new life. Soil is the earth, which supports all living creatures. It is diverse, full of nutrients, such as bacteria, fungi and amoebae, as well as minerals from rocks, including calcium, potassium and phosphorus. Decayed leaves, clay, water and sand provide other minerals like nitrogen and calcium to the soil. All of this enriches the plants that grow.

When you start to view a field in this more complex way, you can see it as a space of potential. The space can become home to different seeds growing into a variety of flowers, plants and trees, just as who you are can become home to a wellspring of experiences stemming from your body, heart, mind and external world. The possibility for growth is always present.

In the mandala of xiu yang you can begin to pay deep respect to the soil that constitutes your personal field. When you begin to show this respect, you see that everything you ingest matters and has the potential to be sacred, in the same way sunlight, soil and rain are sacred to the sprout. What you ingest also has the potential to be profane, damaging, depleting and corrosive in the same way that agents such as salt or chemicals can harm or kill a tree.

Chinese thinkers from ancient times knew this. The fourth-century BCE philosopher Mencius described how 'all things flourish if only they receive their proper nourishment and all will perish if they do not'.[15] In this way xiu yang implores us to remember that diet, thoughts, exercise and meditation do not just keep our body and mind healthy, but allow us to prosper and thrive. These activities nourish the soil that grows who we can become.

Ensuring that the soil of your field receives nourishment is a way to honour yourself and the altar of your field. It is not self-absorbed or narcissistic. It is a gift. When you cultivate your field, you aim to grow the most nourishing and healthy crops. You cultivate yourself to become more clear, balanced and able to live well, to make a difference in your life and the lives of others. With the mandala you are always working to see yourself as part of a greater whole.

By seeing the field of your self-cultivation as a sacred space, like an altar, you can bow deeply to all that is within and around you. You can also begin to care for yourself as part of something greater and more precious, beyond just your personal needs. By caring for and nourishing the soil of your altar you enrich the person you have the potential to become. This is part of the art of xiu yang.

SEEING THE SACREDNESS OF SOIL

The influential Indian philosopher J. Krishnamurti (1895–1986) described how he once took a rock from a garden and placed it on his mantelpiece. Every day he brought flowers to it. By the end of the month the rock became sacred.[16] Anything on which we place our intention and that we appreciate has the potential to become sacred. To understand the metaphors the Chinese drew between the external fields of soil in which we grow and cultivate crops and our own internal field of our self, take time each day to find some actual soil. You can find this soil in a houseplant, park or open field. Take a few moments to look at it, feel the soil with your hands, maybe even smell it. Then imagine that the possibilities latent in the soil are like the possibilities within you to cultivate what brings your body, mind, heart and world greater health, happiness and balance.

CULTIVATING GOOD SEEDS

Given the right conditions, all seeds have the potential to grow. With xiu yang our aim is to grow good crops and keep down the weeds. We can extend this metaphor to many life situations: our thoughts, choices and relationships. Zen monk Thich Nhat Hanh teaches about the idea of good and bad seeds growing in our consciousness.[17] We each have both within us. When we water the seeds that are healthy for us, such as being kind, generous or compassionate, more of these same types of seeds will germinate and grow. Similarly, when we water the seeds of destructive emotions and thoughts, those too can grow and overtake us. If, however, we neglect our good seeds, they can weaken. Thich Nhat Hanh's advice is that we each need a healthy reserve of good seeds to help us through our difficult times.

How do you grow these good seeds and ensure they become helpful resources? You start by remembering that seeds need to grow unseen in darkness before they sprout above the earth. The early stages of self-cultivation unfold in a similar way: much of it is unseen development work that guides you towards becoming a happier, wiser and more fully awake human being.

As you prepare the soil and allow seeds to germinate, remain patient and step back to let the process gradually unfold. Always give your seeds just the right amount of light without overexposing them directly to the sun. Also, create balanced light sources; if sprouts are on a windowsill with only one direction of light, they will start grasping for this light and become what is known as 'leggy' – wispy, thin and weak. When you germinate your internal seeds, remember to give yourself time, space and options for growth. This is often what I tell students who are beginning yoga practice: start slowly and take classes from a few teachers. Try different styles before committing to one path. It is important in the early stages of growth to explore and mitigate the tendency to grasp for results.

Once seeds begin to grow, they require balanced, peaceful conditions. Seedlings are delicate. In Mencius's teachings there is a story about a man who was anxious for his shoots of grain to grow. To make them grow he tried to pull on them, but only resulted in making them wither. He used this story to illustrate that for anyone to become a better person it takes steady work and attention. With self-cultivation Mencius advised that we 'must neither neglect one's shoots nor force them to grow'.[18] If we rush our personal development, we can deplete ourselves or come to resent the results.

This is good advice for any situation, especially when addressing our physical, mental and spiritual development. Take good care of what you grow in the early stages. It can be easy to become overzealous. Enthusiasm can be healthy, but also hazardous. Over the years I have witnessed many students drink the spiritual Kool-Aid and decide to become teachers within one month of practice. Sadly, this often results in physical as well as psychological injury. Yoga, meditation and qigong practices are strong medicine. As blissful as these practices can feel for some, they are also a mirror. Not everything we see reflected back at us is positive or encouraging. Seeing who we truly are through spiritual practices requires courage, the guidance of trusting teachers and the gift of time.

PATIENCE AND STEADINESS

You may not feel immediate results from daily efforts of cultivation. In fact, the effort you put into your daily practice will most likely seem mundane and unglamorous. This is where it can be useful to remember that you can view the ordinary as extraordinary.

Since ancient times xiu yang has involved a healthy amount of discipline and dedication. Exercise, daily routines, sleep cycles, meditation and breathing practices are repeated again and again. Through repetition our effort eventually becomes so seamless that it requires no effort. Within this effortless effort, or *wu wei*, a naturalism arises, which is the essence of the Dao. Just as in the early stages of planting crops when we cannot always see what is beneath the surface, the results of our work come with patience and steady watering and nourishment.

This is demonstrated in how students become masters of Chinese calligraphy. At first glance an observer may see words on a scroll as simple and unimportant. In Chinese culture, however, calligraphy means 'beautiful writing'. It is a high visual art form, surpassing painting and sculpture. How one wrote mattered as much as what one wrote, and what one wrote often reflected the body as well as elements of the natural world. To the calligrapher, writing characters is like a dance: when drawing a line across paper, it is not just the hand that determines the stroke; how the artist shifts their body weight also determines the movement of the brush as it meets the page.[19] As characters take shape, they come to life from the calligrapher's life energy, or qi. Qi has the power to transform a character into natural imagery. The dot of a brush becomes a falling stone, a tiger's claw or an eagle's beak. Characters and lines are carefree or galloping.

To achieve these qualities and master the art of calligraphy, artists repeat the movement of the brush on paper until the process becomes effortless; at this point the calligraphy is executed with perfect, spontaneous form. The same is true with forms such as qigong and tai chi. One stands, moves the body slowly, stands and repeats. Through this repetition a mysterious transformation occurs. The slow movements of qigong can quickly increase energy levels and build surprising amounts of internal heat. The simple process of standing and moving slowly allows space to feel aligned in the body. This opens the lungs and deepens the breathing. As a moving meditation, it calms and stills the mind. It may even change a person's DNA: studies have shown that genes related to inflammation became less active with people who practised regular tai chi or qigong.[20] This is how something ordinary such as writing becomes extraordinary.

Meditation is perhaps the most extraordinary example of what can happen with the very mundane, ordinary act of sitting quietly. If you watch your breathing for fifteen minutes in meditation, you can often feel bored. This is because breath is not nearly as enticing as the distractions of your mind, spinning out memories, stories and elaborate fantasies. Yet the mere process of sitting down to observe the breath again and again has been shown in studies to change brain chemistry as well as the level and state of awareness. It calms and stills the mind. This is an extraordinary process, especially given how busy and distracted our minds tend to be.

To practise xiu yang we must persevere like farmers waiting for crops to bear fruit. In Buddhism this forbearance and patient endurance is known as *khanti*. In the fast-paced, quick-results world of today, slow and steady may seem a thing of the past. Remember, however, that every moment we practise is a reward. As Donna Farhi wrote in her book, *Bringing Yoga to Life*, 'The moment we sit in quiet self-reflection, slowly stretch our limbs, or enter deep relaxation, we become the thing that we are seeking, and in doing so it is possible to experience the end result from the very beginning.'[21]

The neurological and muscular sophistication enabling you to move, breathe and have a conscious, thinking mind is nothing short of a miracle and a mystery. If you slow down to fully appreciate each moment, you may see you are part of a greater and far more powerful force of continuity and life. You are a field: rich, latent and profound in its dynamism. When you remember this, you may experience what the ancient Chinese seemed to know: the return to the innate, ordinary nature, which is an extraordinary oneness of the Dao.

PRACTISING SEEING THE ORDINARY AS EXTRAORDINARY

Sit down for a few minutes and sense into your body. Close your eyes. You may notice thoughts, sensations and experiences. Then open your eyes to take in the richness of colours, textures and shapes around you. Ask yourself: how do my eyes see what they see? How does my consciousness know what is here? How is it we know things and feel conscious? Is knowing ordinary, or is it the result of something mysterious and extraordinary?

STAYING OPEN TO THE LANDSCAPE

Cultivating your fields of body, mind, heart and world means being willing to see the entirety of your personal experience and looking deeply at your own circumstances. It asks you to include the whole landscape and remain receptive to life during the easy and carefree chapters as well as during the heart-crushing episodes. This means staying open to what you resist. This is important but very difficult. Most of the time, when things are hard, we tend to naturally avoid these situations or shut down.

Practices like yoga, qigong and meditation can be useful: they create space for us to feel what we feel and meet the movements of our body, mind and breath as they arise. We become focused inwardly and sensitive to more than just our thoughts. When you do these practices, you embrace a more complete self, and learn to feel everything more fully, including the things you push away. Over the years, staying open to what I dislike has taught me that I do not always have to run away from discomfort or dodge uncertainty, which was my habit growing up. Whenever anyone in my family would fight, I would run to my bedroom and close the door. I disliked confrontation so much that I avoided it whenever possible, including in my relationships and later in my marriage. What I have learned is that this tendency has led to more trouble than good! By gradually accepting confrontation and discomfort I have begun to see that facing my fears also frees them up, and allows me to feel everything – the pain but also tenderness, honesty and joy – more fully.

Staying open to the landscape means meeting many wrenching but invaluable moments of struggle without closing others out or shutting ourselves down. This can become a powerful antidote to cynicism and selfishness. Rather than sink into the murky waters of your personal problems, you can learn to stay standing on steadier ground and more connected to everything and everyone around you. From this position you can fertilise important seeds such as compassion, thoughtfulness and care in your life.

To cultivate the source for happiness, commit to seeing what the Daoists called the 'ten thousand things'. This includes everything between heaven and earth – the joys as well as the sorrows of life. To stay open to all that requires more than just 'thinking' your way through resistance. We can easily become lost in the labyrinth of rumination and thought. Instead of being lost, however, remember that you have a map. The mandala of xiu yang will help you see yourself as more than your thoughts. It helps you keep in perspective that you are a part of an infinite matrix of experiences formed through body, mind, heart and world.

As you journey through the map of xiu yang, remember that, at each turn, you are cultivating and nurturing your heart (*xiu xin yang xin*). The practices, ideas and processes offered in the following chapters are invitations to support the wholeness and balance of nature that is also who you are. By sowing the seeds of greater health, balance and happiness within the sacred fields of the mandala, your heart will naturally become more calm, peaceful, loving and radiant.

PART 2

Xiu Yang
for a Healthy and
Harmonious Body

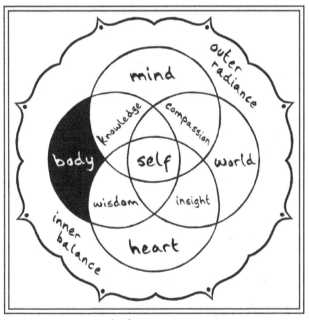

mandala of xiu yang

Many of us feel that our bodies are far from ideal. In fact, they're often a source of frustration: they get sick, feel tired, tight, heavy or are otherwise somehow imperfect. Xiu yang and the Dao teach us that everything is relative and part of a wholeness that is always complete. This includes our bodies. To start the journey into the terrain of a happy and harmonious body, consider seeing your flesh and blood as an innate part of the balanced, natural world. When you feel your body as a source of dismay or displeasure, it signals something has happened to create imbalance and the illusion of separateness. To help you remember and feel the completeness of who you are as part of nature, start by understanding that your body can be like soil. Like soil, it has the potential to be neglected and over-tilled, but equally can be replenished with nutrients and become a source of fruitful bounty.

THE CHINESE APPROACH TO THE BODY

Chinese medicine's approach to health sees the body as comprised of life energy, or qi. Everything – our blood, organs, bones, tissues and nerves – are part of interconnected systems that store and move qi. Since ancient times the Chinese medical approach to health emphasised that healing the body starts with healing the flow of qi circulating throughout the body.[22]

Qi can be a tricky principle to understand and conceptualise, but in the simplest definition it is the energetic blueprint giving life to all matter. In dense forms qi becomes solid matter; in more rarefied or light forms it is breath, ether, the sky and heaven. In our body it is an organising force governing development and growth.[23] It is like the human genome – a vibrant design enabling an embryo to grow and our hearts to start beating on their own. It is in our breath, bones and blood. It animates our every movement, thought and emotion.

Because of qi's universal presence, the traditional Chinese approach to the body is quite different to Western medicine. The Chinese see qi as the force that determines a dynamic interplay between a number of organ and meridian systems comprising us as a whole (meridians are believed to be rivers of energy that relate to organs and flow through your body). In classical Chinese medical theory bone density is determined and affected by the level and quality of qi stored in the kidneys. In conventional Western medicine no such relationship exists.

In the classical Western approach to the body, anatomy and physiology are seen as distinct disciplines. Anatomy, which means 'dissection' in Greek, is the study of the structure and parts of an organism. Physiology, which draws from the Greek word *physis*, meaning 'nature' or 'origin', is the study of the functions within living organisms. Though trends in Western medicine are beginning to shift this perspective, for many years standard anatomy textbooks, such as *Gray's Anatomy*, defined the skeleton as the structure and part of the organism that was seen as separate from the function provided by our tissues, blood and organs to keep us alive. Now, there is an understanding that your bones, for example, play an important role in your immune system by regulating your body's response to invading bacteria and viruses.[24]

Chinese medicine sees blood as the vehicle moving qi through to the organs and meridians. When the flow of blood is healthy and strong, organs are enriched with vibrant, healthy qi. If the flow of blood is erratic or sluggish, qi flow can also become excessive or deficient, leading to stagnation and poor function in the organ systems.

In the yogic tradition, there is a similar concept to qi: *prana*. *Prana* is also defined as life energy, or life force. The difference is that *prana* is not seen to have connections to the organs, elements or times of day. *Prana* moves through the body as different winds, or *vayus*. These winds can also directly affect our health. Having a healthy flow of *prana* is the primary purpose for many who practise yoga postures. For yogis breath control is called *pranayama,* and was the defining practice of physical yoga before modern Western influences placed preference on physical postural practice.[25] When your pranic flow is healthy, you tend to experience stronger digestion, immunity and mental clarity. When it is erratic, low or too powerful, it can affect these functions and disrupt your health.

Whether it is *prana* or qi, each person has a life energy

universally present within them. Your body is the source and foundation for enhancing your quality of life. The overall state of your well-being is dependent on whether your qi and pranic flow is healthy or unhealthy. It is also why so much emphasis in Chinese medicine, Daoism and modern yoga is placed on caring for and cultivating your body and mind to the best of your ability.

4

Living by Our Body Clock

臟腑 學說

We start the journey of xiu yang for the body by aligning certain rhythms with the patterns found in the natural world. Traditional Chinese medicine doctors, Daoists and Confucian sages saw these rhythms operating at three basic levels:

- **DAILY** – the times when you get up, eat, work, rest and sleep can affect your body's overall health.

- **SEASONAL** – how you organise your life seasonally can balance or disrupt your basic well-being.

- **LIFE CYCLES** – gracefully meeting your age and life cycle can mean a more harmonious relationship to how you grow, mature and age.

According to Chinese medicine, you have twelve main organs with corresponding meridian systems relating to certain hours of the day. During these times specific organ systems function optimally. The natural and biological rhythms outlined in the clock are believed to help you regulate your energy flow. It corresponds to and supports two main cycles in your day:

- **YANG CYCLE:** An outward, expansive cycle that is characterised by activity, such as growth, planning, digestion and elimination.

- **YIN CYCLE:** An inward, receptive cycle that allows for filtration, restoration, protection and maintenance.

When you live according to the body clock, you align with this balance of yin and yang, which is believed to be an innate part of your natural constitution.

Following the Chinese body clock is one of the most simple, direct and immediate ways to impact your health and well-being. For example, if you are someone who tends to skip breakfast,

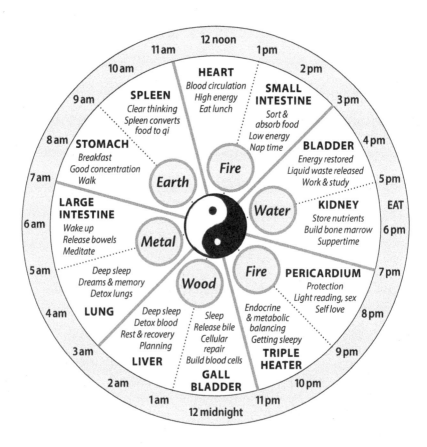

Source: www.fiveseasonsmedicine.com

cultivating the habit of eating a full, hearty meal between the hours of 7 and 9 a.m. may improve your metabolism and overall digestion, circulation and immunity. This is because the food we take in through our stomach in the morning starts to fuel the production of qi, or life energy. The other organs are dependent on this energy to perform their functions and give you the energy needed throughout the day. In my twenties and early thirties, before I learned about Chinese medicine, I would usually sleep late and occasionally skip breakfast. Once I adapted my life more to this body clock and began to get up early and eat a large breakfast every day, many of the digestive disorders I struggled with, such as constipation, bloating and burping (burping is known as 'rebellious qi' in Chinese medicine!), started to fade. As these shifted, I also began practising qigong – a Chinese energy-cultivation art – which has significantly improved my health. We will look more at qigong in the section on balanced exercise in Chapter 6.

THE CHINESE FIVE ELEMENTS

In order to work best with the body clock, it is useful to know that the organs and meridians found in Chinese medicine correspond to different elements and seasons. In total, there are twelve main organs, five elements and five seasons, each with specific emotions and characteristics that manifest when in or out of balance. Understanding the connections between the organs, elements and seasons will help highlight the advantages of following the body clock. The chart overleaf shows the relationship between organs, elements, seasons and their related qualities, emotions and tendencies.

Element	Season	Organs	Quality	Emotion	Responds to	Challenged by
Wood	Spring	Liver and gall bladder	Expansion and growth	Anger	Rhythm, dreams, visions, clear plans, growth	Authority, restriction
Fire	Summer	Heart, small intestine, triple heater, pericardium	Supreme sovereign, separating pure from impure, protection, regulating relationships	Joy	Stimulation, intimacy, love, connection, play	Boundaries, solitude
Earth	Late summer	Spleen and stomach	Concentration, transformation and digestion	Empathy/sympathy	Mother, security, stability, sympathy, understanding	Obsession, stagnation
Metal	Autumn	Lungs and large intestine	Inspiration and letting go	Grief	Father, respect, acknowledgement, warmth	Perfection, the past
Water	Winter	Kidneys and urinary bladder	Flow, reserve and storage	Fear	Stillness, reassurance, wisdom, peace	Flow, the unknown, fears of the future

50

XIU YANG FOR A
BALANCED, HEALTHY DAY

Here is a breakdown of how you can cultivate a healthy structure to your day, and why you might want to choose to do certain activities at these times. By living in closer harmony to this clock, you will orientate towards balance. You can also impact your well-being in tangible ways that nourish and grow solid foundations for health.

3–5 a.m.: Lung (Metal Element)
– Be in deep, restful sleep

If you were in a yoga ashram or living in an Asian temple, you might be up doing breathing and meditation practices at these times. Many nuns and monks around the world choose to rise during these hours. According to Chinese medicine, however, these early-morning hours are the optimal time to detoxify our lungs and be in the final stages of deep sleep.

The lungs in Chinese medicine relate to inspiration as well as letting go. Think about when someone surprises us with a gift: we gasp! Wow! Ah! Our spirits are lifted, and we take a quick, inspiring inhale. When something is heavy, or we feel burdened, we often breathe out a sigh. At this time we ideally allow the lungs to help us with these processes to keep us unburdened and open to the inspirations of the day ahead.

5–7 a.m.: Large Intestine (Metal Element)
– Wake up and eliminate waste

This is the ideal time to rise and begin your day. In Chinese medicine, the large intestine is responsible for transporting and eliminating waste as stools. Between these hours of the day it is therefore a good time to have a bowel movement and release the previous day's digested waste. In letting go, you also make room for the new to come in – be it new food, new experiences or new ideas. Letting go is not always easy. For example, constipation is a common and difficult disorder associated with holding on. As your body's qi and energy begin to find greater balance through a combination of diet, exercise, breathing and daily schedules, these types of imbalances can begin to normalise.

7–9 a.m.: Stomach (Earth Element) – Have a light snack, limit stimulation, do exercise and then eat a hearty breakfast

Once the lungs have been purified and cleansed, it is an ideal time of day to do some meditation and breathing practices followed by mild exercise. Because exercise requires qi, it is best to have a cup of tea or hot lemon water as well as a piece of fruit to start your day.

In the hours between 7 and 9 a.m., your stomach's hydrochloric acid is most effective. This means your digestive juices are strongest. If you eat a full meal each morning you will maximise your digestion, absorption and healthy metabolism. The stomach is the organ that absorbs the foods we take in, breaking them down to be sent on as nourishment to the body. Without the qi from our food the other organs struggle to perform their jobs. Cultivating the habit of eating a large meal at this time will ensure your stomach has sufficient resources to transform qi into the energy you need to get you through the day. We will look at the types of foods that may be best for you seasonally and constitutionally in Chapter 7.

In Chinese medicine the stomach is also an organ that is constantly churning and digesting all that we ingest as life experience, such as our thoughts and emotions. It is a good idea to keep mental and emotional stimulation to a minimum during these hours so as not to overwhelm the stomach's processing, knocking it off balance. Speaking less (or even being totally silent), meditating and doing mild exercise, such as qigong or gentle yoga, during these hours will also support the stomach's ability to digest well.

9–11 a.m.: Spleen (Earth Element)
– Apply mental focus and concentration

The spleen's role is to take the food digested by the stomach, convert it into qi, and circulate it throughout your body. Without a substantial breakfast you may find you have less to distribute. This leads to imbalances in the spleen but can also disrupt the flow of energy to your whole system.

In Chinese medicine the spleen houses something called *yi*, which is best understood as our intention and thoughts. These hours of the day are therefore the optimal hours for undertaking focused mental work, such as studying, writing, organising or researching. When the spleen is healthy, you tend to have clear, undistracted thoughts. When out of balance, you can brood, worry, fret or obsess. Because human beings tend to overthink and be ensnared in stories about past or future concerns, your spleen and *yi* can often feel overwhelmed and burdened. One of the best ways to keep the spleen in balance is embodiment through meditation and movement-based practices such as yoga and qigong. These bring the mind home to the felt sensations of the body, which is the perfect antidote to a troubled mind.

11 a.m.–1 p.m.: Heart (Fire Element)
– Do some active work and then eat lunch!

After a brisk walk or other physical activity, eat a full lunch to feed and nourish the heart's efforts to provide you with energy and nutrition for the afternoon. The heart is described in Chinese medicine as the supreme ruler or sovereign of the body. In China the sovereign is the emperor or empress who governs and oversees the happiness, health and well-being of the state. The heart's job is therefore like the sovereign's: to maintain peace and harmony by ruling with wisdom, insight and benevolence.

Because the heart's main job is to pump blood through your cardiovascular system, maintaining good circulation during these hours is advised. This can be an ideal time to do more active work following the concentrated work of the spleen. The only exception to this would be if you suffer from heart disease or high blood pressure. Because the heart is working at its maximum to circulate blood, too much physical effort during these hours can harm the heart. With heart conditions it is best to rest during these hours to ensure the heart's work is most effective.

1–3 p.m.: Small Intestine (Fire Element)
– Rest, nap, read or do everyday tasks

After your lunchtime meal, it's best to take a rest or do easy errands and tasks that do not require much mental processing or exertion. This is because the small intestine is working to separate the pure from impure. It sends the impure through the large intestine as waste, and sends the pure to the heart (xin 心 – which is also known as the mind in Chinese) so it feels cleaner and brighter. Like any filtration process in which undesirable objects are removed by absorption, it is best to allow the process to unfold without disruption. If the filtration process is incomplete, it can risk contaminating that which we hope to keep pure. For the body this process requires a calm environment for the maximum benefit of filtration to be achieved. When the small intestine is working well, the heart and mind flourish on clear, calm, balanced thoughts. When out of balance, however, your heart and mind can be confused, overwhelmed or unable to make good judgements.

3–5 p.m.: Urinary Bladder (Water Element)
– Have some tea! Also, do light work or complete jobs
that require mental concentration and focus

This is teatime in the United Kingdom as well as in many Asian cultures. This is because the bladder hours are when liquid waste is expelled and your body releases toxicity. By drinking more water (or tea!), you actively replenish your reservoirs and aid the process of detoxification. As waste is removed, some energy in your kidneys is also restored. This can result in a slight boost of concentration or productivity towards the end of the afternoon.

Because of today's hectic lifestyle and increased levels of stress, many of us may not feel this boost. Instead, we may feel depleted and fatigued. This is because the kidneys and urinary bladder store and help regulate our constitutional qi, which is called essence, or *jing*. If you feel tired during this time of day, it is best to rest rather than plough through demanding work.

5–7 p.m.: Kidney (Water Element) – Do some mild exercise that helps improve bone density, and then enjoy a light evening meal

As the energy of the kidneys is most active during these hours, you may wish to do some moderate exercise that increases bone density, such as standing qigong forms that use tensional integrity (placing a combination of tension and compression on the muscles and bones) or weight-bearing exercises from yoga poses, such as locust, downward-facing dog or plank, that move the body against gravity and are believed to strengthen the bones.[26] If you go to a gym, this could also be a good time to practise light weightlifting.

Eating a light meal after exercise will also keep the kidneys' essence, or *jing*, strong. You have two kinds of *jing* stored in the kidneys: ancestral *jing*, passed down from your parents, grandparents and ancestors, and post-natal *jing*, which is what we acquire in life through diet, exercise and lifestyle. Both are believed to support and enrich bone marrow, which is important not only for your basic body structure but is also related to important functions such as building your immune system.[27]

7–9 p.m.: Pericardium (Fire Element) – Spend time curled up with a good book, non-violent movie or loved ones

For these hours of the pericardium (a membrane surrounding the heart), try to cuddle up with someone or something you love, find time for quiet sitting, or enjoy some inspiring and heart-warming reading. Your pericardium is your heart protector. The heart is so important in Chinese medicine, and any direct blow to it would be too painful, dangerous or even lethal. It is therefore the job of the heart protector to keep the heart safe and protected. If attacked by heartbreak, grief or violence, it takes the first blow. In this way it helps deflect tension and keeps the heart from direct injury. Like a good bouncer at a nightclub, however, it also lets in what feeds and nourishes the heart, such as tenderness, kindness, care and love.

In classical Chinese medical texts and Daoist manuals, the pericardium hours are an ideal time for making love. If you are trying to conceive a child, it is thought to be an optimal time to make love. If you are not in a relationship, it can be a wonderful time to be with your pets, friends or other loved ones.

9–11 p.m.: Triple Heater (Fire Element) – Take a bath or hot shower and go to bed

Many of my friends like to have a joke with me and my husband, referring to us as 'Grandma and Grandpa Deemer'. This is because on a number of occasions we have asked if we can eat early and get to bed by 9.30 p.m., which is our ideal bedtime. Going to bed at 9.30 p.m., however, is not always possible given the demands of the modern world. Late working schedules, devices that keep us up, or good late-night television programmes incentivise staying up late. This was certainly true for me until I began to recognise the benefits of an early-to-bed schedule.

The triple heater is like the body's thermostat. Its function is to regulate our temperature in three main areas: the abdomen, solar plexus and chest. These areas are connected by fasciae, or a web of connective tissue. When the temperatures in these three areas are regulated, your body finds homeostasis, or balance. This helps regulate functions such as metabolism, hormone production, mood, reproduction, sexual function and sleep. To help keep your triple heater functioning well it is best to go to sleep during these hours. If you do not get to bed during these hours, you can potentially thwart your body's ability to manage and modulate these activities, leading to problems in circulation, respiration, digestion, elimination and reproduction.

11 p.m.–1 a.m.: Gall Bladder (Wood Element) – Sleep and let your body repair itself

These hours correspond to a delicate time of transition between yang and yin cycles. It is a time when your body begins to restore blood and repair cells, which is a function of the gall bladder and liver. Your liver (the largest organ of your body) and gall bladder (a small pear-shaped organ just under the liver) are both located on the right side of your torso beneath the ribs. In Chinese medicine the gall bladder governs judgement and decision-making. It implements ideas and plans created by the liver. If you are awake during these hours, you may impair your gall bladder's good decision-making, and interrupt its other function of removing and storing bile from the liver. If this happens, it can result in 'too much gall' – which often leads to being rude, impatient and brash or brazen.

Many people today stay up quite late. You may be one of them reading this book! Our devices and habits of watching late-night programmes or other entertainment can be enticing. In Chinese medicine if you are up between the hours of 11 p.m. and 1 a.m., you may increase tendencies towards irritation, anger or even violence. Interestingly, the US Bureau of Justice Statistics reported that between 2002 and 2008, alcohol-related violence peaked at 1 a.m., and, in 2013, the US Federal Bureau of Investigations also reported that the highest incidence of crime in the United States happens between midnight and 12.59 a.m. – a time of night that the body clock advises we should be safely in bed and asleep.[28]

1–3 a.m.: Liver (Wood Element) – Be in deep sleep; time to detox and enjoy dreams that inspire your visions, goals and plans

During these early-morning hours, the body releases toxins that are absorbed by the liver and filtered out as bile to the gall

---

57

bladder. These toxins can be from chemicals or hormones in the food you eat as well as poisons from alcohol and pesticides. To be effective the body should be resting during these hours to ensure a thorough process of absorption and release. If you are awake during these hours, it can negatively affect your liver, leading to increased toxicity and disruptions in other functions governed by the liver, such as menstruation, sleep patterns, hormone production and overall energy levels.

In Western medicine the liver has many functions, including storing sugars and releasing them in the middle of the night. This is why you can sometimes wake up in the middle of the night after eating late, heavy meals or sugary snacks close to bedtime. If you already have glucose in your bloodstream from food, the liver's additional release may jolt you awake. It is therefore a good idea to eat before 7 p.m., and avoid late-night snacks.

A healthy liver also works to support your vision, goals and dreams. This time of night is when some of these dreams may manifest. The liver also works to take in and release anger, which is the emotion associated with the Wood element. An imbalanced liver can lead to irritation, anger or, when deficient, meekness and the inability to stand our ground. A healthy, balanced liver, however, allows you to express anger creatively and constructively in ways that do not blame yourself or others. For example, you can put your anger towards reforming social injustice instead of being frustrated at yourself or your partner when they forget to stir the porridge and it burns.

Final thoughts on time of day

An early-to-bed-and-early-to-rise routine can be the start to supporting and cultivating a healthy and balanced body. While some of these timings of activities may be impossible for you to implement straight away, remember that any seed of change can be planted and start to grow over time. To begin you may wish to set some intentions to change certain patterns, such as your morning or evening routines. Then when these feel anchored in your daily regime, slowly shift your resources to meet other possibilities in how you organise your day. There is no rush. Take your time to explore how the changes feel.

XIU YANG FOR LIVING SEASONALLY

You can also explore adjusting your annual activities according to the Chinese seasonal calendar. In ancient times many Chinese people lived according to an agricultural cycle, where seeds were planted and grown in the spring and matured in summer. By late summer, fruits ripened and bounty was enjoyed, and by autumn there was a harvest. In winter the ground lay fallow and rested before the start of spring's expansion and renewal. You can follow the rhythms of the seasons in a similar way.

Here is a suggestion for how you may wish to view these cultivating activities and priorities according to the seasons:

Spring – Wood Element phase

Start implementing plans and visions for your year. This is a time of year for rising energy. Sow the seeds of new ideas that you wish to undertake, or begin to consider how different dreams you have can be realised. This can be a productive, busier time of year. Watch out for signs of irritation or anger, though, as the emotion of wood is anger. As you begin to expand your vision, plans may not always go as you wish. When efforts are curtailed or plans thwarted, it can be easy to become frustrated, angry or simply to give up. If you sense wood's anger, call on the resourcefulness of trees, which often see objects in the path of their growth and simply grow around them. Remember to stay flexible and adaptable through the spring.

Summer – Fire Element phase

Begin maturing the plans you made in spring, but also start to appreciate the work you have put in to cultivate what you now see growing. Summer can be a time of openness, connection, laughter and fun. The emotion related to summer is joy. The longer days and warmer weather naturally awaken the divine spirit, known as *shen* in Chinese medicine. *Shen* is what animates life, bringing qualities of laughter and joy to the way you live. Enjoy time for play and holidays. Also, remember that the Fire element and summer season relate to the heart. In Chinese medicine the heart does not do well when overstimulated, which can actually result from too much joy. The heart thrives best when calm and tranquil. Give yourself time to be leisurely and relaxed.

Late Summer – Earth Element phase

Late summer is a time when the temperatures are not yet cool but no longer so hot. It is often when the fruit of trees begins to ripen and fall off. Late summer is a time of abundance, transitions and steadiness. Take time to feel nourished and supported by your spring plans having matured through the early summer. If you have had time off over the summer, ease your way slowly back into productivity. Transition your children back into school with earth's steady support. Feel the centring and steadiness of the earth to help anchor you so that you can nourish and care for yourself and those you love.

Autumn – Metal Element phase

Autumn is a time to slow down, be inspired by life, and gracefully and naturally start to let go. As the days begin to cool and daylight hours start to shorten, complement this time of year by also beginning to do less. Just as trees begin to lose their leaves, see what you can pare back in your life. In this process you may begin to see what is of real inspiration and value in your life. This is what often happens when you clear out clutter from your house, or reduce the amount of unnecessary busyness in your life: you see what truly matters and appreciate this deeply.

Winter – Water Element phase

In the winter trees often draw their resources from the branches and leaves to their root systems, which are drinking up precious nourishment in preparation for the growth of the spring. As humans, we can also learn to shift our energies in the winter from outward busyness and activity towards inward rest and stillness. This is not often easy, though, as our society expects us to remain productive 100 per cent of the time. In Chinese medicine, however, this is the time of year to lie fallow. Befriend silence, and listen to the body and mind's need for recuperation and restoration. In this way, you can prepare yourself for the growth and dynamism of spring.

XIU YANG FOR OUR LIFE CYCLES

In a similar way to energy shifts within a day and throughout a season, you can also learn to shift and attune to the different rhythms and activities throughout a lifetime. Throughout history practitioners of xiu yang believed that if people cultivated the right lifestyle from birth to death they could live well into their ninetieth or even hundredth year. Living the 'right lifestyle', however, is understandably hard to attain for many of us given the stresses, uncertainties and demands of our lives. By adjusting one's energies, curtailing negative experiences and embracing self-cultivation practices, they believed everyone could experience a centenarian's life.

Birth to 20 years of age:
Wood Element years

The energy of this time of our lives relates to rising yang, or a time of rapid development. It is when we experience exponential growth. Our bones and bodies develop, we expand into our ego and personality, and our minds fill with visions and dreams.

20–40 years of age:
Fire Element years

This is the time of maximum yang, when our bodies no longer grow but our hearts mature. Ideally, this is when we begin to deepen our connections to our work, life and family. If you can orientate towards cultivating a healthy, balanced heart, especially during these years, your capacity for compassion, kindness and love can increase and become more radiant.

40–60 years of age:
Earth Element years

After the peak of your maturing fire decades, earth years are when you can ideally find some equilibrium in life. This means there is less overall striving to do in your work, relationships and family, and there is more time to enjoy the fruits of life and abundance of living.

60–80 years of age:
Metal Element years

This is a time in life when you can have a stronger connection to spirit and letting go of what no longer serves you. It is a time of refinement and appreciation. It is also when you can cull what is unnecessary so that deeper meaning and value in life are revealed.

80–100 years of age:
Water Element years

In China age is celebrated, because with it comes the experience gained from wisdom. Water is associated with deep knowing, insight and listening. Others look up to us for our life experience. Others listen to us because we know how to be still and listen to them deeply. In this time of life, be willing to meet the unknown and welcome the mystery.

5

Breath and Longevity

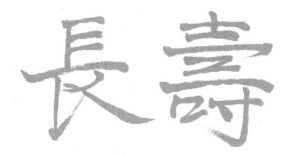

The field of your breathing requires steady, daily cultivation. The bounty you reap from the regular tending to your in breath and out breath can not only bring you a healthier and more balanced body but also unlock what the ancient Chinese sages believed was the gateway to longevity.

Breathing is the first and most prominent practice outlined in the fourth-century BCE text, *Inward Training (Neiye)*, believed to be the oldest mystical Daoist text. Breath is said to bring us back into the state of oneness with the Dao – a quality that is always available but sometimes lost to us because of 'sorrow, happiness, joy, anger, desire and profit-seeking'.[29] If we cast these qualities off, our mind returns to a state of equanimity. The process of casting these off is through accruing the benefits of breath, described here as a process of coiling, contracting, uncoiling and expanding:

> *Considering the practice of the Dao,*
> *You must coil, you must contract.*
> *You must uncoil, you must expand.*

You must be firm, you must be dedicated.
Guard aptness and do not become lax.
Abandon the excessive and discard the trivial.
When you reach the ultimate limit,
You will return to the Dao and inner power.[30]

The wisdom from these ancient manuals offers us a connection back to what people thousands of years ago valued: breathing your way to living a long, healthy, meaningful life.

REDISCOVERING AND REFINING OUR CAPACITY TO BREATHE

Breathing is a natural, ongoing process that keeps us alive. Yet in many classes I teach, from yoga to meditation and qigong, I have often had students confess that they are confused about the breath, and do not know how to breathe properly. Many of us may have lost our inborn capacity for deep, nourishing and regenerating breath that we each naturally have when in utero or as newborn babies. With some willingness and basic understanding of respiratory functions you can rediscover and refine your ability to breathe. You can cultivate your breath in ways that yield an optimal harvest of life energy, which is qi or *prana*.

Learning how to value and honour your breath can be a tricky process. Breathing happens every moment we are alive, yet most of the time we are unaware and unappreciative of the way breath confers life. Many also develop patterns of breathing that impede the body's capacity for full breathing. Perhaps we have been taught to keep our bellies in and restrict our centre, which forces the breathing into our upper chest rather than in the lower part of the lungs. When we inhale, our lungs can extend all the way down to our waist level at our lower back. When we breathe into this lower area, we use more of our lungs' capacity (normally, we only take in on average 500 millilitres of air, but our lungs can take in as much as 5000 millilitres).[31]

Often, however, stress has impacted our breathing, making it shorter, shallower and quicker.

My breathing has been an ongoing journey of difficulty and discovery. As an asthmatic child who also contracted bronchitis and pneumonia at the age of four, I have struggled most of my life to breathe deeply. When I began practising yoga, and later qigong, I started to recognise an unhealthy pattern of shallow and restricted breath. While I now understand the value of deep breathing, and some of these patterns have reversed, I continue to work on refining and cultivating my breath each day. My asthma, while much better than when I was young, continues to periodically flare up; when it does, I am reminded of how quickly any deep, nourishing breath can fade. In meeting my own struggles to breathe, I have learned that the best way to rediscover and refine the breath is to see breathing as a natural process that can be encouraged to flourish and grow. We can reclaim what lifestyles or illness have taken from us, and begin to breathe as we may have done as a child: free, easy and deep.

CELLULAR BREATHING

Every cell in the body breathes. Every cell also hungers for the steady supply of oxygen that is carried through our blood. Oxygen is delivered to our cells by our in breath. Cells then expect the removal of toxins, such as carbon dioxide, to be granted via the out breath. When the expelling of toxins is complete, each of your cells takes a rest and is momentarily still before starting the process of ingesting nutrients once more. This desire for renewal, growth and rest at your cellular level drives your need to breathe.

Cells begin breathing in the mother's womb. In this state the body floated in fluids, weightlessly drifting and breathing without cares about gravity or the healthy function of the lungs. The way cells breathed was via our mother's umbilical cord: it brought in blood rich with oxygen, and similarly transported out waste.

While in an embryonic stage cells follow a pattern and movement of expansion and contraction: as oxygen and nutrients enter in through a cell membrane, the cell expands. When it discharges carbon dioxide and other waste through the same cell membrane, the cell condenses. After this contraction, the cell momentarily rests before taking in another round of oxygen. Once you are out in the world, your breathing follows a similar pattern. Though the rhythm is different, your respiratory

CELLULAR BREATHING EXERCISE

This exercise can be done first thing in the morning, before bed or in a midday break.

1. Lie down on your back in a comfortable position, knees bent over a yoga bolster or pillow.

2. Notice how your body and breathing feel; this will help you establish a baseline for doing the work. To begin, invite your breathing to move freely and naturally.

3. Next, take a deep breath in and visualise your cells absorbing nutrients such as oxygen through their membrane and expanding.

4. Exhale out a long, smooth breath. As you do this, imagine your cells removing toxicity and waste from the same membrane and gently contracting.

5. Pause gently at the end of your exhale, and imagine your cells at rest.

6. Repeat steps 3–5 for between 5 and 25 minutes, depending on your time availability.

7. Finish by taking a moment to observe how your body and breath feel. Notice any shift or change from when you began.

muscles are designed to create three parts to breathing: inhaling, exhaling and pausing at the end of an exhale. By visualising this process happening within your cells, you can develop a useful blueprint for understanding and creating movement in your body as it breathes.

DISRUPTION OF CELLULAR RESPIRATION

When cellular breathing is functioning well, cells are vital and healthy. When this process is disrupted, cells struggle, function chaotically, and eventually die. One cause of strain and disruption to cellular breathing is mental or emotional tension. When we begin to feel stress, we experience an increased level of a hormone called cortisol in the body.

Cortisol is known as the stress hormone. Each of us needs a certain level of cortisol as it is what lets our body gather physical resources to respond quickly to emergencies and get ourselves out of dangerous situations. It does this by shutting down unnecessary functions such as our immune system, metabolism and the creation of proteins and carbohydrates necessary for digestion and growth (such as bone formation and blood production). If you stay in elevated states of stress and experience consistently high levels of cortisol, your body begins to suffer from these impaired functions. On a cellular level the areas of tension restrict the flow of blood and oxygen, eventually starving cells. On a broad level it weakens and impairs the function of nearly every major system of your body, from your immune system to your heart rate, digestion and elimination. This makes you more susceptible to chronic or acute illnesses, such as infections, heart disease, ulcers, constipation, sleep disorders and anxiety.[32]

Cells may also struggle with muscular tension. When muscles are regularly or habitually constricted and tight, the flow of blood to the cells of that muscle area is restricted, eventually causing the cells to become damaged and unable to perform a healthy exchange of nutrients and waste. If you are someone who spends long periods of time sitting at a desk in a slumped position, the tissues around certain muscles may tighten and harden while others weaken and slacken. Any tightness or contraction reduces the capacity for blood flow, which in turn starves the cells of a healthy exchange of nutrient intake and waste removal. The same is true if you sit slouched in couches or even in rounded car seats: the front of the chest collapses, which affects your pectorals as well as the muscles that flex your neck. All of these muscles suffer as a result of a lack of optimal cellular renewal.

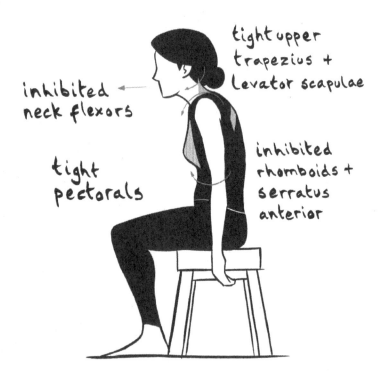

inhibited
neck flexors

tight upper
trapezius +
levator scapulae

tight
pectorals

inhibited
rhomboids +
serratus
anterior

BREATH AND GRAVITY

As soon as we are born and take our first breath, the body starts the complicated process of finding air and nutrients. We are asked to confront two foreign forces: breath and gravity. We start to breathe, suck and swallow, and later begin to crawl, walk and stand. All these actions involve figuring out how to best position our bodies to support the weight of our heads to navigate the world.

To survive and thrive, we have to work out ways to balance these forces. This is one of the primary gifts that movement-based practices such as qigong and yoga can offer you. Because these practices specifically ask you to co-ordinate movement with the breath, you are given an excellent platform to explore this balance.

A TOUR OF YOUR DIAPHRAGM

Taking a tour of your basic respiratory anatomy can help you learn how to cultivate an optimal breathing pattern. Your main respiratory muscle is called the diaphragm. It sits inside your lower ribs. It is located in the mid-to-lower part of the torso. As a result, the main work of breathing is not done in the upper chest, where many of us may tend to breathe. The optimal breath can be felt in your back, sides and abdomen. The diaphragm, which is shaped like a parachute or jellyfish, alternately expands and contracts to draw the breath in and out of the lungs. When you inhale, the diaphragm moves downwards towards your abdomen. It flattens, like a plate. When you exhale, the diaphragm moves upwards, like a closed parachute or umbrella.

The diaphragm is a thick muscle – about as thick as your thumb. Importantly, it stands on two short columns at the back spine. These columns are called the crus. *Crus* in Latin means 'legs'. These legs are tendinous fibres that extend the diaphragm down the lumbar spine. I point this out because when you breathe in and your diaphragm flattens down, the legs of your diaphragm also extend down the lumbar spine. When you breathe out, they relax. In Chinese medicine this area is where your two kidney organs are positioned. It can be a good incentive to breathe low and deep to this area of your back body, as it is believed that your kidneys catch hold of the qi brought in as breath from your lungs and store it for future use.

Equipped with this knowledge of your diaphragm's main movements, try this as a way to begin cultivating a nourishing and deep breath:

1. Choose a comfortable position, either sitting upright or lying down comfortably with your knees bent or placed over a yoga bolster or some pillows for support.

2. Notice your breathing. Is it in the chest? Abdomen? Sides of the ribs? Is it fast, slow? Shallow or deep? Coarse or smooth? Choppy or even?

3. Place your hands on your abdomen. Can you feel the rise and fall of your breath here?

4. Interlace your fingers and rest your thumbs on your belly. When you inhale, expand the palms open towards your abdomen. This is like the diaphragm's movement of opening downwards into the shape of an open parachute or plate. Keeping the fingers interlaced, relax the palms together as you exhale. This is like the shape of the diaphragm relaxing, and a closed parachute or umbrella.

BREATHING FREELY

When you understand the basics of how the diaphragm moves, you can begin to explore natural and free patterns of breathing. In *The Breathing Book* Donna Farhi outlines the basic characteristics of breathing. We have explored one of these characteristics, the diaphragmatic breath. I have based some of the following suggestions on her work.[33] As you read these exercises, feel your diaphragm's organic movements, and integrate the following characteristics into your approach to breathing.

1. **TIDAL MOVEMENTS** – The breath comes in and moves out like the tides of the ocean. Like these ocean tides, a natural breath does not suddenly stop. There is a continuous rhythm, an effortless ebb and flow of each in breath to out breath. Visualise your breath as the ongoing movements of the tides.

2. **RADIAL SYMMETRY** – Breath follows a pattern of moving from our centre to the periphery and back again. As you inhale, feel your centre expand out 360 degrees towards your peripheral body. As you exhale feel the release from the periphery back towards your centre.

3. **LET THE BREATH BREATHE YOU** –The breath is not something that originates from an external source. Your breath is natural, and comes from within you. Feel your breath arising from deep within the chambers of your body as you inhale. Feel it return to this source as you exhale.

4. **INHALE, EXHALE, PAUSE** – Like the movements of our cells which expand, contract and rest, let your breathing move through three parts: inhalation, exhalation and a pause. Extend your out breath, and then linger in the pause. This will let your exhale feel longer than the inhale. Allow the pause at the end of your exhale last longer than you think before you take your next breath in.

5. **FLUIDITY** – Keeping in mind the expression that the only constancy is change, let your breath adapt naturally and fluidly like water to all the circumstances that arise. Some breaths will be longer or shorter, fuller or more shallow. This is like life: our mind, body and emotions reflect our breathing. Allow these changes to arise like the movements of waves in an ocean.

---

6. *WU WEI* – Let your breathing orient towards effortless, spontaneous ease. Let it flow the way a river flows in an ongoing, continuous and unbroken stream.

FIVE CHARACTERISTICS OF HEALTHY BREATHING

These are the five classical methods for breathing that have been used in China for centuries. When our breath matches these characteristics, it can lead to benefits such as lowering blood pressure, slowing the heart rate and the more expedient elimination of toxins.

1. SLOW (慢 *man*). Breathe using a slow rather than hurried, rushed or impatient rhythm. Taking time to breathe opens greater opportunities to absorb oxygen into your bloodstream. Slow breathing also invites your nervous system to become steadier, which can support important functions such as healthier immunity, circulation and digestion.

2. LONG (長 *chang*). Allow your breath to be long rather than short. When you consciously extend your breath, you calm your mind. You also increase oxygenation and toxicity release. Every normal breathing cycle has an inhale, an exhale and a pause. After you breathe in, invite your exhale to last at least two seconds longer than your inhale. Never underestimate the importance of your exhale. When you exhale, you eliminate up to 70 per cent of your body's waste.[34] Rest and pause before starting to inhale again.

3. FINE (细 *xi*). A fine breath is the opposite of one that is rough or coarse. Think of a fine-toothed comb that untangles hair, or a fine sieve or cheesecloth that filters out debris, leaving only what is most pure. This is what we can achieve with fine breathing.

4. EVEN (均 *jun*). Invite your breath to become even rather than choppy. Like the movement of gently rocking waves, let

the tempo of your breath find a rhythm that is smooth and consistent. In creating this consistency, you may get a feel for how your abdomen naturally expands and contracts with each breath.

5. DEEP (深 *shen*). Let the breath be deep rather than shallow. Breathe to the lowest place in your body. As we explored earlier, the lowest parts of your lungs sit on your back body near your waistline and kidneys. Long term, a deep breath expands lung capacity and thereby increases oxygenation and carbon dioxide removal from your bloodstream. It also reduces tightness of the chest, upper back and neck by drawing on the diaphragm and intercostal muscles to breathe, which are our primary respiratory muscles (secondary muscles are our pectorals, scalenes and sternocleidomastoids).

BREATHING:
THE KEY TO LONGEVITY

Just let a balanced and aligned [breathing] fill your chest
And it will swirl and blend within your mind,
This confers longevity.

Inward Training (Neiye), Chapter 21 [35]

For many of China's earliest sages longevity was the primary goal of xiu yang. Chinese medical texts, such as *The Yellow Emperor's Classic of Medicine*, believed that given the right conditions, human beings could live to over 100 years without showing the usual signs of ageing.[36] One of these conditions was the belief that 'respiration was of essence and energy', which helped to keep the spirit in the body, and prevent it from decaying.[37] There is some truth in this, as we have seen: deep breathing feeds our cells, removes toxicity and reduces stress.

When you access this capacity to breathe naturally and fully, you grow vitality and steadiness in your life.

Here are a few exercises you may wish to introduce into your day to help you access the wisdom of breathing your way to a longer, healthier and more balanced life.

THREE DAILY XIU YANG PRACTICES FOR SOWING THE SEEDS OF HEALTHY BREATHING

1. Every day, take a few moments to connect to your breathing. Use the 'Five characteristics of healthy breathing' (see page 72) to observe whether your breathing can lengthen if it is short, slow down if it feels too fast, become more fine and smooth if it feels coarse, more even if it feels choppy, and deepen if it feels shallow.

2. Set an alarm for every hour to remind yourself to breathe diaphragmatically. When the alarm goes off, pause in the midst of whatever you are doing and sense a moving from the centre outwards and back again in your breathing, like the movement of your jellyfish-like diaphragm expanding and contracting.

3. First thing in the morning and last thing before you fall asleep, take a few minutes to notice the process of cellular breathing at work in your body. Let your body breathe while visualising the healing work happening potentially in every one of your cells. Let your in breath revitalise and nourish your cells. Let your out breath release waste and toxicity, leaving the cells resting in a vibrant, radiant calm.

6

Moderate Exercise
for Maximum Health

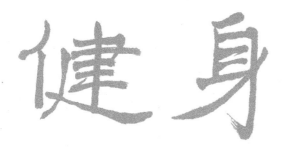

In the West generally exercise is seen as something strenuous, or a means of shaping the body into an idealised version of who we think we should be: thinner, stronger, faster and more fit. I certainly carried this ideal well into my life; I owned an embarrassing number of aerobics DVDs and have rather unsuccessfully tried jogging and working out at a gym. After I started practising yoga, there was a short period of time when I loved to go to the hard classes that made me sweat and ache for days afterwards. I confess that I secretly aspired to achieve what I saw as a perfect 'yoga body': lean, lithe and flexible.

Though some are beginning to see exercise as a system for well-rounded health, notions in the West of a perfectly shaped body remain primarily influenced by the ancient Greeks.[38] They believed human beings could attain a flawless physique and strength resembling the gods they worshipped. Athletes competed at Olympic festivals to prove their abilities to over-come human measures of endurance, power and speed. They used exercise to prove they could be indomitable, independent and more like the gods to which the games were devoted.

The ancient Chinese, however, held a different view: moderate exercise yields maximum health. The second-century AD physician Hua Tuo, who is also considered the father of Chinese medicine, stated that 'the body should be exercised, but not to excess. Exercise improves digestion and keeps the meridians clear of obstructions. In this way, the body will remain free from illness.'[39] Instead of seeing exercise as a way to remould a flawed body into a perfect form, Chinese tradition saw moving, breathing and stretching as a means to rediscover a balanced wholeness. This is a view I have come to appreciate. Just as we would not want to overexpose crops to too much sunlight and heat, we don't want to expose ourselves to excessive exertion.

Many in the health profession are also beginning to recognise the merits of this approach. An article published in 2017 by *Frontiers in Immunology* shows low-impact, mind–body intervention practices, such as mindfulness, yoga, qigong and tai chi, reduce the level of a compound called NF-κB that is activated by stress and responsible for the expression of inflammation-related genes.[40] Research published in 2015 by Harvard Medical School and Beijing University also shows that exercises such as qigong and tai chi help people with a variety of medical problems, as well as preventing the onset of conditions such as high blood pressure, heart disease, diabetes, arthritis and osteoporosis.[41] Of the 507 who took part in the trial, 94.1 per cent reported that tai chi had a positive effect on their overall health. Some of the participants had goals of general health, while 50 per cent sought to achieve better physical balance or prevent falling, which can lead to fractures or other serious injuries for older adults. In a 2016 study participants with knee pain found twelve weeks of doing tai chi was not only as effective as physical therapy for relieving discomfort, but it also led to less depression and had a positive impact on their quality of life.[42]

TRAIN FOR TEN YEARS OLDER THAN YOU ARE

Today, the American College of Sports Medicine advises older adults to undertake mild exercises such as yoga and tai chi to increase strength, improve balance and prevent falls.[43] Why wait, though, until you are older to reap these benefits? With xiu yang you can plant the seeds today to help you create bounty and health in your older years. We can do as my friend Matthew Cohen, founder of Sacred Energy Arts, advises: 'train for ten years older than you are'. At forty-six I can train to support and respect my body for when I reach fifty-six. I love how this perspective invites me to lean into and accept the changes I will naturally undergo as my body ages.

Some may read this advice as unusual, especially since many people feel averse to the notion of getting older. The emphasis in the West for most adults over the age of twenty-five is to feel, act and look younger. To fast-forward your life and think ahead to when you are thirty-five when you are only twenty-five can feel overwhelming and off-putting! Yet there is wisdom in cultivating habits now that will serve you as you age. Hopefully, when you think of yourself in ten years, you will envision yourself as maintaining some strength, agility and health rather than succumbing to depletion, stiffness and disease. To feel this way in the future, you must first accept that as your body ages, it tends to dry up and slow down. Sometimes people forget this, and may inadvertently follow practices that deplete them, leaving them even more dried out and weaker in their older years. By carefully selecting practices with the primary intention of promoting health, balance and long-term sustainability, you can learn to enjoy better physical health and vitality through your older years.

THE TRADITIONAL CHINESE
APPROACH TO EXERCISE

Exercise continues to be seen as a central component of longevity and healing practices in China. Since as early as the fourth century BCE, the Daoist sage Zhuangzi described how practising exercises that mimicked birds stretching and bears hanging nourished the body and conferred longevity.[44] Zhuangzi, known for his elliptical humour and tendencies towards slight exaggeration, once exclaimed, 'I have been cultivating my person for one thousand two hundred years, and my body has never become frail!'[45] Scrolls dating to 168 BCE also show forty-four figures performing animal-like movements known as the *daoyin* (see below). *Daoyin* means 'leading and pulling'. These exercises were described as useful for preventing and curing illnesses such as kidney disease, rheumatism and anxiety. Many of these forms of exercise are still practised today as popular qigong forms known as the Five Animal Frolics and Eight Silk Brocades.

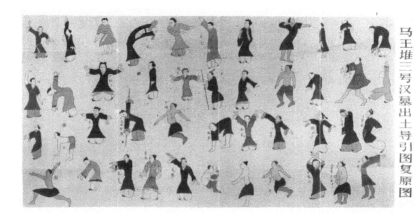

马王堆三号汉墓出土导引图复原图

As a practice of 'leading and pulling', the *daoyin*'s approach to exercise focused on three primary aims. These aims are described by Daoist and Chinese long-life practices expert Livia Kohn in her book *Chinese Healing Exercises: The Tradition of Daoyin*:[46]

- **TO GUIDE AND DIRECT QI.** Guiding your body's qi to be in harmony with the Dao will help you feel the balance and wholeness of yin and yang. This balance aligns you with the energies of nature and the universe.

- **TO PULL ON AND ACTIVATE STRENGTH.** Stretching the muscles, releasing the joints and extending the limbs circulates and moves the qi in healthy ways.

- **TO RELEASE PAIN OR A PROBLEM AND STIMULATE THE BODY'S HEALTH.** *Daoyin* exercises often involved pulling the qi out from a diseased part of the body by lengthening muscles and stimulating meridian lines.

As the seventh-century medical handbook *Origins and Symptoms of Medical Disorders* describes, the *daoyin* therefore 'consists of drawing together in one's body all the bad, the pathogenic and the malevolent forms of qi. Then one follows them, pulls them in, and guides them to leave forever. This is why it is called *daoyin*.'[47]

A CONTEMPORARY APPROACH TO AN ANCIENT METHOD

Compared to people who lived thousands of years ago, we spend more time sitting in chairs for longer periods, often in front of computer screens or looking down at digital devices such as tablets and mobile phones. Our more stationary and sedentary lives may therefore require updated remedies from those who practised *daoyin*. Here are some more contemporary exercises from qigong and yoga that can help cultivate greater health and nourishment in areas of your body that may have become underused or overstretched.

The following three practices are suitable for most ages and fitness levels. The first is a contemporary qigong warm-up. The second and third utilise fluid patterns and combine movements from yoga and qigong, and have similar goals as the *daoyin* of harmonising the qi flow in the body, stretching muscles, releasing joints, decreasing pain and stimulating the body's health.

ARM SWINGS

This tai chi and qigong warm-up is designed to offer a quick and efficient way to circulate qi and improve your blood flow. It also releases tension in the back, chest, neck and shoulders. It can be done anywhere, and at any time of the day. In many parks across China or in Chinatowns in the West, you will see people swinging their arms as a form of self-cultivation! In this popular form of movement, your arms lightly slap against the skin of your abdomen and lower back. This stimulates the function of your digestive, reproductive and respiratory systems, and is generally good for the health of your kidneys. Practise this for between 5 and 10 minutes for optimal health.

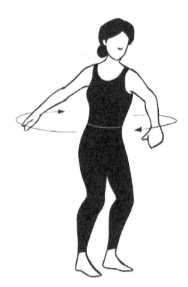

1. Stand with your feet shoulder distance apart and turned straight.

2. Relax your joints and keep a slight bend in your knees. Allow your arms to relax by your sides.

3. Breathe naturally and deeply. Do not be concerned about co-ordinating the breath with the movement. Focus your eyes on the ground in front of you.

4. Root your feet and grip your toes slightly. Keep your knee-caps as stationary as possible throughout this practice, letting the swing move from the torso and hips. Be careful not to twist or strain the knees.

5. Gently begin to rotate your torso towards the left and then the right, allowing your arms to organically swing from the turning of the hips and spine rather than any effort from the arms themselves. As your turns build momentum, the arms will slap lightly against the front and back sides of your lower torso – the abdomen, lower back and kidneys. Continue for between 5 and 10 minutes.

6. Begin to slow the movements down and settle back into stillness. Observe how your hands and arms might tingle with a sense of energy, and how the body feels more vibrant and alive.

FIGURES OF EIGHT FOR THE HIPS, SHOULDERS AND SPINE

This sequence is based on the work of Donna Farhi, who integrates the shape of the figure of eight into many of her movement patterns. By moving our hips in figures of eight we naturally complement the round ball-and-socket joints of the hips and shoulders. This is highly therapeutic for the joint structure but also for the muscles that surround the joints, which can often become tense, rigid and stiff.

In the West the figure of eight is also the sign of infinity, which is a word derived from the Latin *infinitas*: [being] without end. The image of the sideways figure of eight, or '∞', is used in mathematics to represent a number without limit. Its design suggests oneness and wholeness, balance of opposites and completion. It is a pattern found throughout many cultures; renderings of it first appeared in early Indian and Greek art, and in Arabic calligraphy the motif stands for the name of God. For the Maori it illustrates the flow of energy between the physical and spiritual worlds as well as two lives eternally becoming one. For the Chinese it is the same flow as found in the yin and yang symbol.

Interestingly, the figure-of-eight pattern of movement mirrors the way blood circulates through the heart. No one understands the reason behind this pattern, but cardiologists say that when they place a pacemaker into a patient, they know it is in the right position when the wires of the pacemaker physically begin to move in a figure of eight completely of their own accord.

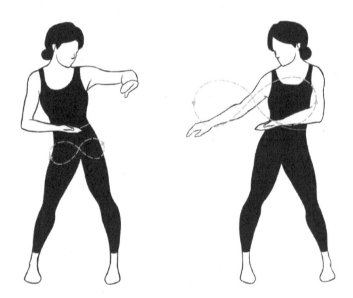

1. Stand with your feet shoulder distance wide, feet turned straight. Let the knees be slightly bent. Relax the arms by your sides.

2. Breathing naturally and fully, begin to circle the hips in a figure-of-eight pattern.

3. After a few minutes, introduce the arm movements; as the hips circle, allow the arms to also naturally start to move in figure-of-eight patterns.

4. As your hips circle to the left, let your hands and arms also move to the left, creating one half of a figure of eight. The right palm will face upwards towards the sky, and the left palm downwards to the earth. This is a variation on the tai chi practice known as silk reeling.

5. As the hips begin to circle towards the right, the arms and hands begin to move towards the right. The right palm will turn to face downwards towards the earth, and the left palm upwards towards the sky.

6. Gently feel the shoulders rolling with this fluid movement pattern of the arms from side to side. Imagine the hands move along imaginary wind or water currents that support them as they glide through the infinity loop.

7. Continue for between 3 and 5 minutes in one direction, and then change directions. You can also do this for longer periods of time, or try a variation with the legs wider apart.

YOGA/QIGONG SUN SALUTATIONS

This is a sequence I have developed and often teach in my vinyasa yoga classes as a way to condition the circulatory and respiratory systems and build strength and integration through the body's main muscle groups. It integrates the more fluid movements of qigong within a mindful flow of movements based on the classical yoga sun salutation sequence, *Surya Namaskār*.

As part of saluting the sun, this sequence involves visualising carrying sunlight in your hands, which can be a source of warmth, nourishment, growth and insight. It involves feeling the earth, horizon lines and movement patterns, such as wind and water, supporting your body. Use organic, fluid, gentle movements. You can repeat this sequence two to three times per day as a way to connect you to the elements of the natural world that feed, inform and sustain us. You may want a yoga mat for this practice, or a sturdy, non-slip surface.

1. **START STANDING:** Breathe with a calm, steady breath. Stand your feet hip distance apart in mountain pose, or *Tāḍāsana*. Bring your palms together in front of your chest into prayer position.

2. **BEGIN THE SUN SALUTE:** Inhale and reach your arms out to the side and then overhead. Exhale and fold your body down towards the earth with the hands together in prayer position. Inhale and lift your head and heart towards the horizon line. You can place your fingertips on the ground or lift your hands towards your shins. Exhale and fold forward.

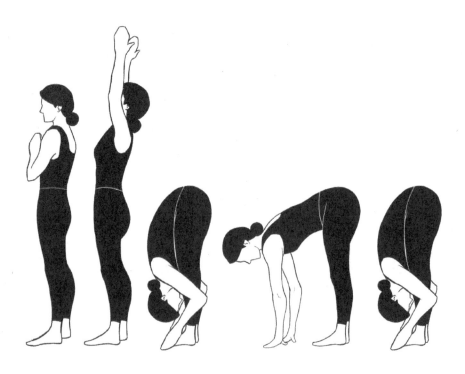

3. DO A 'VINYASA' VARIATION: Inhale and step back, lowering your knees into child's pose on your exhale. Inhale and roll forward to your hands and knees. Exhale, roll the front of your body slowly down to the ground. Inhale into a gentle backbend of either cobra (with your pubic bone on the ground) or upward-facing dog (only your hands and your feet on the ground). Exhale, tuck your toes in, and lift up and back into downward-facing dog.

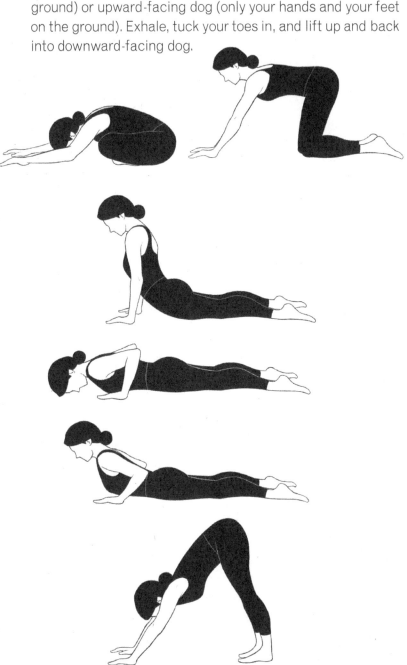

4. PREPARE TO CARRY THE SUNLIGHT: Inhale your right leg behind you into what is called a downward-dog split. Exhale your right foot forward towards your right hand into a lunge, like it lands softly on the moon. Inhale and lift your arms up into crescent pose (*ashta chandrāsana*). Imagine your hands are filled with the light of the sun.

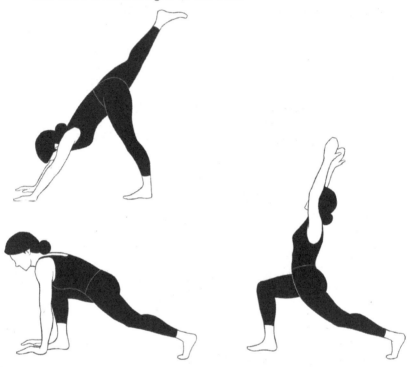

5. CARRY SUNLIGHT IN YOUR HANDS: Carry sunlight around to the back of the mat as you exhale. Imagine the arms move along imaginary wind and water currents to create fluid, unbroken movements. Inhale and lift your arms filled with the light of the sun into crescent pose. Exhale and carry the sunlight back to the front of your mat, again imagining fluid, unbroken movements carried by imaginary wind and water currents. Inhale into crescent, hands filled with the light of the sun, and exhale, lower the hands and step back into downward-facing dog.

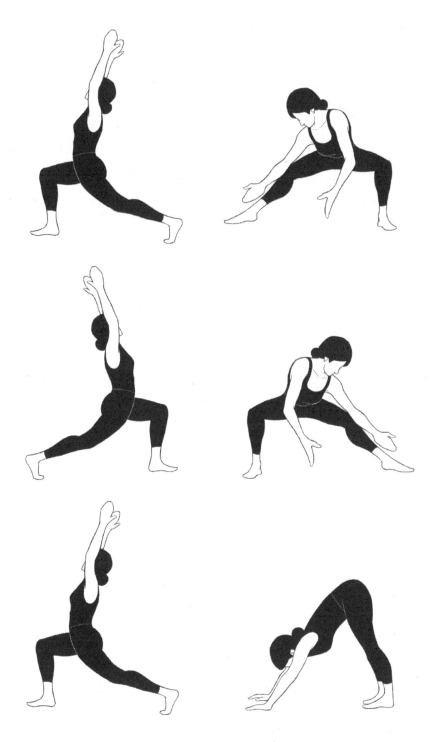

6. Touch the knees to the ground, and repeat the steps on pages 85–87 on the left side.

7. **COME TO THE FRONT OF YOUR MAT:** From downward-facing dog, step or lightly jump the feet forward to the front of your mat. Inhale to lift your head and heart towards the horizon line. Exhale and fold. Inhale and use your arms and hands to gather the sun-warmed earth and lift this towards the sky.

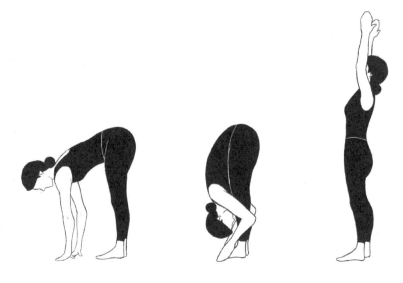

8. **FINISH WITH A QIGONG 'FILLING'.** With the light of the sun you have carried in your hands, exhale slowly and bend your elbows with the middle fingers pointing towards each other. This is called 'filling'. Fill the light of the sun into the form of your body as the hands lower down in front of your face, chest and belly. This qigong practice uses the hands and intention to direct energy, or qi, more specifically into the body for healing.

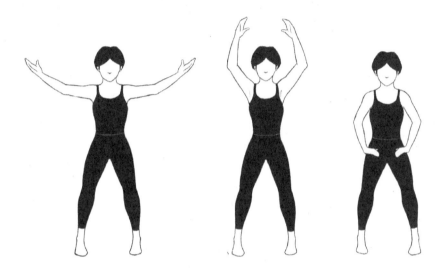

You can repeat this variation of sun salutes between two to three rounds. Upon finishing, notice the effect of the practice on your body, breath and mind.

7

Nin chi le ma?
Have you eaten?

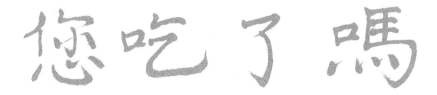

When someone you know sees and greets you, you rarely receive a simple *ni hao* in Mandarin. Most of the time you will be asked, *Nin chi le ma?*, which means, 'Have you eaten?' I have always loved this greeting as it reflects both the central importance of food to Chinese culture as well as how the Chinese have traditionally gauged one's general state of well-being based on whether or not they have been fed. If someone has eaten, this means they are well; if they haven't, then something may be amiss.

The close connection of food to health has a 3000-year-old tradition. *The Yellow Emperor's Classic of Medicine* states: 'disease of the spleen corresponds to a yellow and sallow face and one should eat salty foods to help dry [the body's] dampness, such as black beans and soybeans, pork, chestnuts, and the leaves of a bean plant'.[48] The reasoning behind this is that food has always been a source of qi, and therefore considered medicine. Recipes for dishes were similar to those for medicines. In China today there are thousands of recipes to treat conditions ranging from a common cough to hypertension, insomnia, tumours, frostbite and diabetes.[49]

Diet therapy is therefore one of the staples for cultivating and maintaining good health. Our dietary habits can affect the direction and quality of our energy flow. How, when, what and the environment in which we eat can all influence the stability and vibrancy of our body's qi.

While this may seem complicated or unusual to many people living in the West, every Chinese doctor will tell you that when you cultivate a balanced, positive attitude towards food, you will not only become healthier but enjoy your food, satisfy your hunger more quickly and prevent weight problems. The xiu yang of diet for a healthy and harmonious body asks that we place importance on the quality of food we consume, the quantity we eat, and how and when we eat it. Understanding the potential of the healing qualities of food and how you consume it enables you to take another step towards finding a natural equilibrium of health and balance.

THE IMPORTANCE OF WHEN, HOW AND HOW MUCH

Have you ever wondered how much food is actually a healthy amount? In our culture we often receive conflicting messages around this question: rail-thin models suggest we should restrict what we eat, but most food advertisements tempt us with mouth-watering bites of bliss into foods we know will tip the calorie counter far past its peak.

The classical Chinese perspective held very specific opinions on the subject of food quantity, and warned about the consequences of either over- or undereating. Chapter 23 of *Inward Training* tells us:

> *Considering the way of eating,*
> *If you over-indulge, your qi will be injured.*

This will cause your body to deteriorate.
If you over-restrict, your bones will be weakened.
This will cause your blood to congeal.
The places between over-indulgence and over-restriction,
We call this 'harmonious completion'.
Here is the lodging-place of vital essence.
It is also where knowing is generated.
When hunger and satiation lose their regulation,
You must make a plan to rectify this.[50]

The wisdom in these words may strike you, as they did me when I first read them: no one wants to cause their body to deteriorate or face their blood congealing. What the ancient Chinese knew is that there is a balance in how you can approach food that starts with changing your tendencies and habits of eating. When you do this, you will naturally move towards 'harmonious completion' or a healthy balance to your diet.

The most positive and influential change you can make towards cultivating a balanced approach to food is paying closer attention to *when and how much* you eat. These two factors play as much of a role in healthy digestion as *what* you eat. From personal experience, on days when I eat a heavy late meal before going to bed, I often wake up feeling tired and foggy-headed for much of the day. If I eat a light meal at least three hours before bed, I sleep better and often feel energised the next day. This knowledge has been insightful, but also highly rewarding: I can regulate my energy without having to significantly change what I eat.

Food is becoming more closely associated with the causes of illness and disease: too many sausages and other processed foods can cause cancer, while lactose- or gluten-free diets have offered life-changing solutions to people who cannot digest dairy products or who suffer from coeliac disease. What you eat can directly affect your health. As the impact of industrially farmed meat on the environment deepens, and increased awareness about animal welfare intensifies, diet has also become an expression of ethics. This is in part why I like the quote from *Inward Training*: it remains impartial on these fronts and refrains from telling us what or what not to eat; it simply suggests that we should have a plan to neither overindulge nor over-restrict. This, the ancient authors say, is the key to balance.

Here are four ways that can help you cultivate a more balanced approach towards your diet *without* having to radically change what you eat:

1. **EAT BREAKFAST LIKE A KING, LUNCH LIKE A PRINCE AND DINNER LIKE A PAUPER.** In other words, eat the largest meal of your day at breakfast and the smallest at dinner. For years, I ate in the complete opposite order: a tiny breakfast, big lunch and even bigger dinner. Though eating this way is not always possible when in social situations, at home I try to stick to this plan. My breakfasts are enormous – often I will eat sourdough toast, vegan cheese, seeds, porridge, and occasionally eggs. My lunches are also substantial, but for dinner I prepare something light: stir-fried vegetables or soup with fresh bread. These meals are surprisingly satisfying and filling, and eating light dinners has had a positive effect on my sleep quality as well as metabolism and appetite.

2. **TAKE TIME TO PLAN AND PREPARE YOUR FOOD.** Foods are often packaged or prepared. Preparing food yourself gives you time to think about the process of feeding your body the most qi-rich and balancing experience. As you plan your meal, be realistic: good meals do not have to involve extensive shopping lists or take a long time to prepare. An easy stir-fry of tofu and green beans can take five minutes. A simple broccoli and potato soup can take ten minutes to make. A steamed sweet potato and black bean dish can take fifteen minutes. Of course if you have more time, slowly cooked foods can be a pleasure to prepare and watch as they transform. As you chop and sauté, savour the colours, flavours and smells of your dish. This will connect you more

to the source of your food, and also give you more control over the ingredients you include.

3. **EAT IN PEACE**. When I worked in journalism in China, I often scheduled lunch or dinner meetings. If eating alone, I would also read or watch movies while I ate. Sometimes (and still, occasionally, I confess), I scroll through social media feeds on my phone. According to Eastern approaches to health, we should create a distraction-free space to appreciate and give full focus to our meal. Distractions such as using phones or checking emails as we eat can deter the smooth processing and integration of the food we consume. I always notice how much less satisfying a meal is and how my digestion feels more sluggish if I have been distracted while eating. As much as is possible, leave the phones behind as you enjoy your meal.

   Also, try to let meals be a time spent with friends, family and loved ones. If you live alone, let time spent eating be a quiet time for yourself. Leave business and important or emotional talks for another time. Tension, deliberation and too much thinking can burden the stomach and spleen, which blocks and weakens our ability to digest food. This can result in a loss of appetite, bloating or stomach pain or digestive disorders. How you feel as you eat will affect how your body digests and transports qi from food. Therefore, take your meals in as leisurely and relaxed a way as possible.

4. **EAT SLOWLY AND MODERATELY**. Every organ in Chinese medicine has a storage and supply of qi. When you chew your food slowly and thoroughly, the Chinese medicinal opinion is that this supports your spleen organ's qi, which satisfies your hunger more quickly and prevents obesity.[51] If you swallow your food and do not chew it fully, you not only tend to overeat but also feel sleepier and more bloated after you eat. This is because after large meals, the body draws the qi and blood into the centre to digest the excess. If you regularly overindulge, this can impair your digestive

organ function and lead to health problems in digestion and elimination, respiration and circulation. Try chewing each bite of food 20–30 times. This will mitigate the problems and tendencies to overindulge and tax your body's ability to digest.

From a Western perspective, chewing not only breaks down the food, making it easier to digest, but we also release saliva. According to the American Dental Association, saliva contains enzymes that aid in digestion and makes food easier to swallow. It also washes away food and debris from the teeth and gums, releasing substances that prevent cavities and other infections, and providing high levels of calcium, fluoride and phosphate ions that keep the surface of your teeth strong.[52] Eating slowly also makes you feel fuller sooner; this is because it takes the brain approximately twenty minutes to send out signals that you are full.[53] Chewing is a mechanical part of digestion; when you chew fully, this gives your organs less work to do. When food is broken down more before swallowing it, we increase the surface area of the food and extract far more nutritional value from what we eat.[54]

When you eat more slowly, you also develop mindful attention. This attention helps you attune to the flavours and textures of your food, but also invites a deepening appreciation and awareness of where the food has come from and how it has been produced. Zen Buddhist teacher and poet Thich Nhat Hanh refers to mindful eating as an opportunity to remember what he terms 'interbeing': when we eat a piece of bread, we remember that the grain has been grown by the sun and nourished by the rain and earth. What you are eating, therefore, is not just bread but what has been grown by sunlight, rain and soil.[55] Knowing this can help you remember that we are made from and are part of the elements of the natural world.

FOOD AS MEDICINE

The traditional Chinese understanding of food as central to balance and health began in the Zhou Dynasty (1046–256 BCE). Since then, food types, flavours and colours were believed to affect organ function and disease. *The Yellow Emperor's Classic of Medicine* advises: 'the pungent flavour goes into the respiratory tract; when there is an illness in the respiratory tract one should not each too much pungent food'.[56]

Today, this legacy continues. Certain foods continue to be used to help cure illnesses or treat qi deficiency, stagnation or 'rebellious qi', which is when qi flows in the opposite direction to its normal flow. Food can also be used to enrich the blood, treat the spirit, or regulate the bodily fluids. Physical and emotional disorders were also believed to be caused by factors such as wind, cold, dampness, heat and dryness, and could be treated by nutritional therapy. There are also certain foods that Chinese practitioners advise should be eaten during certain seasons of the year or during certain times of your life.

Foods can be classified into five energetic categories of hot, warm, neutral, cool and cold. Hot foods tend to activate and mobilise energy. Warm foods strengthen yang energy and qi. They also warm the body and organs. Neutral foods build up qi and stabilise the body. Cool foods tend to slow down qi and clear heat. Cold foods tend to cool internal heat and calm the spirit. This classification is based on 3000 years of application, observation, experience and intuition.[57]

The temperature classification given to foods reflects whether they fall into a yin or yang category, and can likewise affect one's overall constitution. The methodology behind diet therapy is nuanced and complex, but a general approach is that you should eat all five ranges of food in balance, with certain foods eaten more in certain seasons (see pages 101–2 for a guide to seasonal eating). If you tend to burn hot or have excess yang energy, you would be advised to eat cool or cold foods, and if you tend to feel chilly and sluggish, which are signs of excess yin energy, you might be advised to eat warm or hot foods. Individual adjustments to a diet can be made based on the season and determined by any pre-existing diseases or conditions.

Overleaf are some examples of foods based on their temperatures, from Joerg Kastner's book, *Chinese Nutrition Therapy*.[58] While these foods can be prescriptive, it is always best to consult with a trained traditional Chinese medicine doctor before making significant changes to your diet. They are also guidelines, and not meant to infer that you must eat certain foods to feel a certain way. These categorisations do not take into account your personal medical history, allergies or ethics around eating meat or types of sourced foods, which certainly play important roles in how many people today choose to eat.

If approaches to diet therapy are of interest to you, please see the Additional Resources at the end of this book.

EAT THE FIVE FLAVOURS
(*WU WEI* 五味)

In addition to knowing that certain food groups can be used to balance your body's constitution and maintain health, you can also consider integrating these approaches into cultivating a healthy approach towards what to include or aim for in your daily diet. In *The Yellow Emperor's Classic of Medicine* we are advised that foods come in five flavours: sweet, sour, bitter, salty and pungent.[59] In the text each flavour is related to specific organs and their associated colours[60] (see page 100).

The five flavours are the oldest system of food classification. Though prescribed as remedies or balances to many health conditions, in general eating a balance of these five flavours as well as colours in your meals can support a healthy and balanced flow of qi through your body's organs and meridians.

Food examples	Cultivation in the body	Cultivation in the mind	Good if you …
TEMPERATURE: **Hot yang**			
Grain alcohol (made from corn, yeast, sugar and water, in low quantities), lamb, and spices, such as cinnamon, garlic, ginger, curry, paprika and pepper	Increases energy, aids digestion, good for feeling cold, boosts immunity	Mobilise energy, uplift	Feel cold and have poor circulation, have chronically cold hands and feet, feel low energy or depressed
TEMPERATURE: **Warm yang**			
Chicken and beef, salmon, coffee, red wine, butter, goat's cheese, fennel, peach, leek, onion, and spices like rosemary and basil	Warms the body, improves intestinal function, warms and strengthens the triple heater, good to treat symptoms from colds, such as runny nose, chest cough etc.	Stimulation and creativity, invigorates thought	Feel tired, tend to get sick often
TEMPERATURE: **Neutral**			
Honey, cow's milk, cheese, eggs, carrots, cauliflower, figs, plums and potato, corn, lentils, millet, peas, rice, spelt and hazelnuts	Stabilises and harmonises the body	Harmonises mental and emotional states	Have problems maintaining energy levels

Food examples	Cultivation in the body	Cultivation in the mind	Good if you ...
TEMPERATURE: Cool yin			
Salt, soy sauce, prawns, bananas, oranges, tomatoes, watermelon and spices, such as dandelion	Soothes the body, supports fluids and blood, slows down excessive energy, clears heat	Regulates overstimulation and overthinking	Burn hotter and have dryness of skin, feel restless, anxious, tend to speak loudly
TEMPERATURE: Cold yin			
Black teas, fruit juices, peppermint, wheat beer, tea and soya milk, yogurt, celery, cucumber, soybeans, spinach, courgettes, tofu, barley, wheat and spices, such as tarragon	Creates cold and cools internal heat	Calms the spirit	Have night sweats, hot hands and feet, hot flushes, are quick-tempered, have difficulty sleeping

Flavour	Organ and element	Colour	Effect in balance	Effect in excess
Sweet	Spleen and Earth	Yellow	Warms and nourishes body	Leads to phlegm build-up and flesh, obesity
Sour	Liver and Wood	Green	Soothes heat and emotional stress and anger	Damages muscle tone and can negatively affect rheumatism and arthritis
Bitter	Heart and Fire	Red	Supports digestion, calms mental strain	Dehydrates and overheats the heart; inhibits the spirit
Salty	Kidneys and Water	Black	Cools, moistens and loosens, aids in digestion	Dehydrates, hardens muscles and damages bone
Pungent	Lungs and Metal	White	Moves qi, increases circulation and loosens stagnation	Causes dryness and restlessness

EATING SEASONALLY

Our bodies are affected by changes in temperature, light and the energetic traits of each season. When you introduce ways to eat according to these seasonal shifts, you can also begin to align more closely with the rhythms and cycles at work in the natural world.

SPRING: This is the time of year when yang energy rises. It is characterised by growth, expansion and vision. As spring is associated with the organs of the liver and gall bladder, eating foods that supplement these organ functions can be beneficial, such as sour flavours, green vegetables, mildly warming foods.

SUMMER: Summer is the season of maximum yang. It relates to the element of Fire, which corresponds to heat and upwards movement. Bitter flavours and cooling foods are best to eat during this time of year. Also, fruits and raw vegetables can be consumed in the summer. Think salads and fresh lemonade!

LATE SUMMER: This is not technically a season, but in the Chinese Five Elements theory there is a fifth season related to the Earth element. It is a time of year that comes after the heat of summer and before the coolness of autumn. It usually begins in early-to-mid August and ends in mid-to-late September. During this time of year avoid greasy, excessive dairy and sugar: these obstruct the spleen's healthy function. Stay away from too many raw and cold foods. It can also be good to eat neutral foods as well as orange- and yellow-coloured vegetables and fruits. Make sure to eat plenty of grains, which are considered sweet, such as rice, corn, wheat, barley and rye.

AUTUMN: In the autumn, the earth begins to cool down. It is the time of yin rising. As a result, pungent, warming foods that make up for the cooler temperatures are advised. Start to season your meals with more garlic, chilli, ginger and onions.

These will help to build what is called your *wei qi*, or defensive qi. Your *wei qi* is believed to be located beneath the surface of your skin, and helps protect the body from external harm, such as viruses and bacteria.

WINTER: Winter is the time of maximum yin. It is also when you are most susceptible to colds and viruses. To counteract this it is advised to eat more salty and sweet flavours as well as warming or hot food. Be careful not to eat too many hot foods, though, as these can dry up your body's fluids and deplete your yin resources.

PART 3

Xiu Yang for a Balanced Mental and Emotional Life

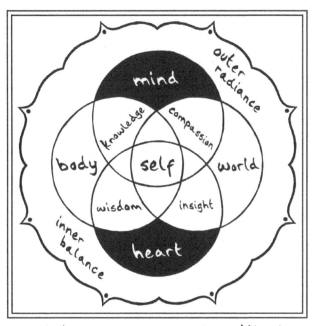

mandala of xiu yang — self-cultivation

What is a balanced mental and emotional life? What does it look like? In science balance is defined as a state of equilibrium, where all forces are cancelled out by equal, opposing forces. Equilibrium is a state where no one thing is stronger or greater than another.

If we applied this definition to our mental and emotional lives, chances are we would become extremely boring human beings! We would not love, feel pleasure, excitement or anger at injustices. We would never let thoughts build into ideas, visions and dreams. Everything would end up being placid and flat. Is absolute balance something that we can or should cultivate in our mental and emotional life? Probably not. What we can work towards with xiu yang for our mind and emotions is a balanced *response* to whatever is arising in our experience.

Looked at from this perspective, to be 'balanced' is more in line with homeostasis, a state that implies a *tendency* towards balance and equilibrium that requires constant adjustments to help regulate this state. When the winds of life knock you off your feet, you get back up more quickly. You may feel angry, but do not stay angry for days, weeks or years. You may have your heart shattered into a thousand pieces from a break-up or loss, but do not stay heartbroken for thirty years. Rather, you respond to your heartbreak and gradually open to the possibility of loving again and meeting someone new in the coming years.

On the map of your mandala finding balanced mental and emotional states falls into the domain of xiu yang for the mind and heart. What are the best tools to help you meet the complications of having a thinking mind and feeling heart? Sitting down quietly, experiencing your own consciousness more clearly, and connecting to your deeper knowing. This process of self-cultivation is the art of meditation.

8

Meditating on the Breath

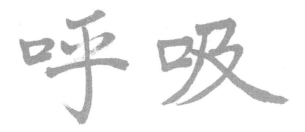

Breath is so ordinary that we usually overlook it. Sensory stimulation and an active mind often mask awareness of simple, moment-to-moment processes like the body breathing. Yet in many spiritual traditions, from yoga to Daoism and Buddhism, the breath is the starting point for focusing the mind and softening the heart. This is because unlike other unconscious activities, such as our heart beating or digestion, breathing is the only activity that will happen unconsciously which we can consciously change at will.

In Chapter 5 we explored the importance of our breath for the health of our cells and overall physiological well-being. In this chapter we will consider another equally important role that the breath plays in the cultivation of ourselves, which is its relationship to our thoughts and emotions. By incorporating xiu yang practices of breathing meditation you can learn to embrace the spirit and mystery of life simply and naturally unfolding, which is not unlike the simple and natural way in which plants grow and flowers blossom. Breath awareness also cultivates essential skills to meet obstacles to this simplicity with more spaciousness and ease. With patience and practice meditative breathing can help you attain the positive forces of mental and emotional health, happiness and balance.

THE MIND IS A MUSCLE
– BREATHING PRACTICES FOR
CONCENTRATION AND FOCUS

Meditation is a training of the mind and heart. When you practise breathing meditation, you begin to train your mind to stay present and focused. Just like you might train a muscle to become stronger through weightlifting or other exercise, the first stages of meditation involve training the mind to become stronger. A stronger mind here means one that is less distracted and more able to concentrate and be calm. Concentration and a feeling of calm allows you to become more centred and relaxed – two things that are not often easy in our busy and distracted lives.

SITTING UP OR LYING DOWN?

When practising meditative breathing, it is best to sit upright with your spine straight. If sitting on the ground, use a few blankets, a yoga bolster or *zafu*, which is a round meditation cushion. If sitting on the ground is difficult for your knees or back, or if you have a physical disability or are less able-bodied, sit on the front edge of a chair with your knees bent at ninety degrees and your back straight.

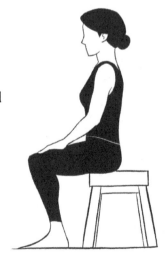

If you wish to practise breathing meditation while lying down, it can feel comfortable but also make you sleepy. If you choose to lie down, place a pillow or yoga bolster under your knees for support and a folded blanket or low pillow under your head. This will relax your neck and lower back. To help you stay awake rest your elbow on the ground while lifting the forearm and hand of one arm upright so that it is perpendicular to the ground. If you start to fall asleep, the arm will begin to flop and wake you up.

COUNTING BACKWARDS

This breathing meditation practice is one I learned from Erich Schiffmann, who was my first yoga teacher. His approach let me start and maintain a consistent meditation practice during the first few years of learning to sit quietly. It is included in his book *Yoga: The Spirit and Practice of Moving Into Stillness*.[61]

The practice involves a simple focus that builds the muscle of your mind. It takes about eight minutes to do. You will count backwards from the number fifty to zero. Count the odd numbers on your inhale, and the even numbers on the exhale. Throughout the practice let your breathing be natural and relaxed. Rather than control the breath, allow it to come in and out normally. As it flows freely, you can learn to move out of the way of the breath and open more fully to an experience of simply sitting quietly and being still.

There are three stages of this practice:

- **FROM FIFTY TO TWENTY.** Exhale and mentally say 'fifty'. Then inhale and say 'forty-nine', and exhale 'forty-eight' and so on. Do this until you reach the number twenty, and exhale.

- **FROM TWENTY TO ZERO.** Once you reach twenty, only count the even numbers. This means for the number nineteen, do nothing; then exhale and mentally say 'eighteen'. Inhale and do nothing; then exhale and mentally say 'sixteen'. Do this until you reach zero.

- **BEYOND ZERO.** When you reach zero, stop counting, but continue to breathe naturally, just as you were doing when counting the breath. Continue to watch the breath and sense its natural incomings and outgoings. Sit as still as you can without feeling stiff or rigid. Relax into the stillness.

As you do this practice, you may notice thoughts and distractions arising. You may also notice that the mind becomes engaged by something else, and you lose track of the number you're on. If this is the case, simply start again from fifty and count down again.

While some practices of meditation and yoga are aimed at a cessation of thoughts (the *Yoga Sūtra of Patanjali*, for instance, defines yoga as the restriction or stopping of the busy mind[62]), the aim in this meditation is not to prevent thoughts from arising or to block them out. Rather, breath becomes a backdrop against which you notice your thoughts. This builds staying power in the mind. As you notice thoughts coming in and out, simply do your best to let them go and come back to the breath. In the next chapter we will explore some techniques that can help you meet your thoughts and respond to them with greater skill, insight and wisdom.

CULTIVATING MINDFUL BREATHING

Cultivating mindfulness of breath is not a breathing exercise. It is one way you can focus and direct your mind. It is a reminder of the changing nature of all experience. With every inhale experience arises; with every exhale experience dissolves and fades away. If we are in harmony with the changing tides of our breath, we can begin to align with what the ancient Greek philosopher Heraclitus (540–480 BCE) observed: 'nothing is permanent but change'.[63] When we make peace with change, we see that whether it be pleasure and joy or sadness and pain that arise in our experience, awareness and calm are also possible. Breath is one of the best ways we can cultivate this possibility through developing a conscious and more intimate relationship with what is always present yet never the same.

The Buddha taught conscious and mindful breathing as the first step in meditative focus. He spoke about this in a sermon called the *Ānāpānasati Sutta*, or 'Mindfulness of Breathing'. This is also outlined in the text, the *Satipaṭṭāna Sutta*, or 'Foundations of Mindfulness'. The emphasis given to the breath reflected his belief that when you learn to breathe with awareness, gentleness and compassion, you have an opportunity to step more fully into the present moment and awaken from the onslaught of stories, thoughts and compulsions that ensnare your heart and mind.

The Buddha described how the development and pursuit of mindful breathing bears 'great fruit'.[64] What are the fruits that we enjoy as a result of our efforts of cultivation? Insight, wisdom, compassion and – ultimately – liberation from our everyday burdens of confusion, unhappiness and pain. Breath helps you remember your innate ability to find true peace and calm abiding in any moment. It wakes you up to your true nature, which is a connection and oneness with all things.

The teachings on mindful breathing offer us a simple path to find this awakening by helping us come back to the present moment. In the words of Insight Meditation teacher Joseph Goldstein, mindful breathing 'is the antidote to distraction and discursive thoughts'.[65] By focusing on the breath mindfully our busy mind starts to settle, which helps us feel relaxed and more peaceful.

While extensive instructions on breathing can be followed (for example, the *Ānāpānasati Sutta* offers sixteen stages of practice), there are four preliminary instructions on breathing that can help you drop a solid anchor into a daily breath-focused self-cultivation routine.

THE FOUR STAGES OF MINDFUL BREATHING, AS TAUGHT BY THE BUDDHA[66]

1. *As you breathe in, say to yourself mentally,*
   'I know I am breathing in.'
   As you breathe out say,
   'I know I am breathing out.'

This may sound simple, but the mind tends to pull away quickly and find more interesting topics on which to focus, such as memories, plans or stories. Noticing when the mind pulls away is part of the practice of mindfulness. Each time you notice your mind somewhere other than the breath, gently pivot and reorientate it back and begin breathing consciously again, repeating this mantra.

2. *Become aware of the length of your breath. If you breathe*
   in a long breath, know you are breathing in a long breath.
   If you breathe a short breath, know you are breathing in
   a short breath.

I like this approach because it tells us that any kind of breath is good; we do not have to make it a certain way. It simply asks you to become aware of whether the breath is long or short, and know it as such. This helps you relinquish your efforts to control the breath. It reminds you that mindfulness of breath is not a breathing exercise, but rather a practice of becoming aware of your experience of the present moment. It is beginning to sensitise you to the ordinary process of breathing, but with more subtlety and focus.

3. *Breathing in, I practise experiencing my whole body.*
   Breathing out, I practise experiencing my whole body.

In this third stage, we begin to shift from knowing the breath to an experience: the practise and cultivation of the breath. With more intentionality behind your practice of mindful breathing you can begin to deepen your awareness of the breath as it moves through the sensations and terrain of your body. As this happens, you begin to feel the breath more intimately. You also begin to sense the effect your breath has on your body. When you inhale, where does the breath go? Does it move outwards, downwards, backwards or sideways into the chest and abdomen? When you exhale, what are the areas of your body that soften and relax? Beginning to feel how and where your breath affects your body can help refine and sharpen your relationship to breathing. You can begin to step more fully into the flow of sensations, and ride the breath as it ripples through you.

4. Breathing in, I practise calming the body.
Breathing out, I practise calming the body.

This fourth stage helps you calm your breath, body and mind. When the breath is calm, the body relaxes. As the body relaxes, the mind quiets down and becomes more still. Likewise, as the mind quiets, the body relaxes, and the breath becomes more peaceful. The breath therefore becomes an agent of cultivating ease. In this stage the Buddha teaches that you can begin to glimpse the feeling of being aware but also more awake and insightful. This state was the basis and springboard for the Buddha's own awakening. It can also be yours through steady practice.

THREE HELPFUL TIPS FOR MEDITATIVE BREATHING

1. *Let the breath be natural and free.* Remember: meditative breathing is not about regulating or controlling the breath. It is about letting go of control. Celebrate and embrace the changing nature of each breath.

2. *Practise becoming still.* Familiarise yourself with the actual feeling of stillness and peace.

3. *Train your attention to stay.* One of my favourite meditation cartoons is of two dogs sitting on the ground on yoga mats with a bowl of incense sticks in front of them. One dog looks at the other and says, 'The key to meditaion is learning to stay.' When your attention strays, come back. Return gently and deliberately and as frequently as is necessary to the sensations of your breath.

WALKING MEDITATION WITH BREATHING

Another very effective way to practise mindful breathing is to do these practices while walking. Concentrating on the breath and number of steps immediately shifts the focus of your mind away from tendencies to contract and tighten around difficult experiences to something immediate, such as your legs and feet moving. I remember once, while hiking up the side of a very steep Alpine mountain with some friends, I became deterred. I was tired, sweaty and out of breath. I thought about stopping and resting, but my friends were far ahead of me, and I didn't want to fall too far behind. As I continued hiking up the slope, judgements ganged up on me and spat at my mind: 'I should do more cardio exercise. My lungs have always been so weak. They must think I am a princess. I should have known better than to go hiking today.' Then I remembered the practice of walking meditation and breath. I counted my steps as I breathed in, and counted my steps as I breathed out. Inhales were four steps, exhales were six. Before I knew it, I was at the top of the slope. My body felt light and invigorated.

Perhaps you have had a similar situation unfold, where a tendency to be in your head becomes a hindrance to your ability to act. The next time thoughts try to invade your mind, try walking meditation, and see if it helps you come back to the present moment and release the chokehold of negative thinking.

WALKING MEDITATION GUIDE: As you walk, count three, four or five steps with your inhale. Do the same with your exhale: count the steps you take. Walk steadily and naturally. There is no need to slow down your gait or control the shifting of your weight. There is also no need to control the breath. Sometimes your breath may cover more steps, sometimes fewer. Simply witness how many steps accompany each breath.

STANDING QIGONG MEDITATION

When we stand and meditate, we can feel the whole body included in our experience and awareness. This standing practice was taught to me on a windy day by Sifu Matthew Cohen. It uses the image of the roots of a tree growing wide and down deep into the earth for steadiness, stability and nourishment.

ROOTS TO THE CENTRE OF THE EARTH

As in other meditations, allow the breath to be natural and relaxed.

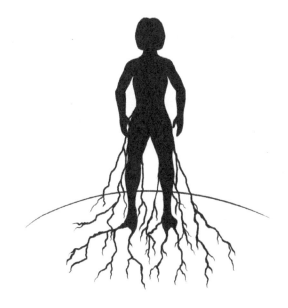

1. Stand in *Wuji*, or Emptiness Stance, which is the qigong standing position. For *Wuji* let the feet be shoulder distance wide and turned straight. Keep the knees slightly bent and the joints of the body relaxed and open.

2. Take a few breaths into your lower *dantian*, which is an energy centre located in your abdomen, a couple of inches beneath your navel centre. It is where qi is believed to be stored, cultivated and refined.

3. Inhale and begin to visualise your breath extending from your *dantian* down your legs, through your feet, and into the earth like the roots of a large tree. Let the roots move out wide as well as deep down towards the centre of the earth. Exhale and let the roots stay in the earth while simultaneously drawing nourishment from the roots back up into your *dantian*.

4. Repeat this, letting each breath extend the roots of your imagined tree deeper and wider into the earth with each inhale. With each exhale, invite the nourishment from the earth to feed and replenish your *dantian*, which can store this energy and use it to help improve the circulation and function of your body's energy.

5. To start, stay with this visualisation for 3–5 minutes. As you become accustomed to standing for longer periods of time, you can do this for up to 20 or 30 minutes.

> *If you can be aligned and still*
> *Only then can you become stable.*
> *With a stabilised heart-mind at the centre,*
> *With the ears and eyes acute and bright,*
> *And with the four limbs firm and fixed,*
> *You can make a lodging place for vital essence.*
> *The vital essence is the essence of qi.*
> *When qi is guided, vital essence is generated.*
>
> Inward Training (Neiye), Chapter 8[67]

Remember that meditative breathing is never an escape from yourself. It is a way into the present moment of experience through consciously becoming aware of something always available: the breath and sensations of your body. This gives you the space to begin cultivating your capacity to quiet the mind. It allows you to let the busyness of everyday life settle. In this space you will find more awareness, insight, compassion, wisdom and awakening.

9

Mindfulness: Cultivating Skilful Responses to Life

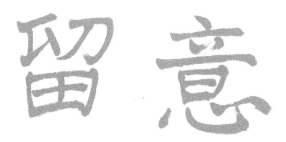

When we lose our balance in life, our response is not always graceful. We easily feel disparaged, confused or blame our hard-luck story on ourselves or others. Feeling this way can be exhausting. Our reaction to feeling knocked down may also be to distract ourselves with other things that bring momentary relief, such as food, alcohol or drugs. Sometimes we bottle up our emotions because they are too difficult to accept, or unintentionally end up hurting those we love.

This is all normal. What mindfulness offers you in these situations, however, is a way to bounce back with more grace. It gives you resilience and the gift of responsiveness, which is what helps you stand back up on your feet when the winds of life blow you off-centre. It gives you tools to keep the awkward, unskilful or detrimental tendencies to react to difficult situations in check. For these reasons it is one of the most effective, practical and transformative means to practise xiu yang for your mind and heart.

WHAT IS MINDFULNESS?

Though a popular catchphrase today, mindfulness is a technology that has been around for thousands of years. It is a practice developed by the Buddha 2600 years ago to help people ease their hearts and minds and relieve the burdens of delusion and pain. The original word used for mindfulness in Pali, which was the language of the Buddha, was *sati*. *Sati* means to remember, recollect or have in mind. What you are guided to remember is your capacity to guard the mind and heart against unhealthy and destructive tendencies, and to be present in a way that is compassionate and responsive instead of damaging and reactive.

Mindfulness is also a practice of seeing and freeing. It invites you to begin tracking the subtle yet sticky filters of clinging and pushing away that lead to suffering. When you become aware of these, you are given skills to disentangle yourself from the destructive tendencies of your mind and emotions. These skills support your ability to differentiate between healthy ideas – such as clear, kind, compassionate thoughts – and the 'weeds' of worry, anxiety, doubt, judgement or fear growing in your heart and mind. If you regularly uproot the corrosive weeds of your thoughts and emotions before they invade and overtake the open field of mental and emotional life, you can steadily begin to nurture what supports your long-term happiness, health and balance. You will also witness more wholesome mind-states that are guided by knowledge, compassion, insight and wisdom – the qualities that transform us at a deeper level. In time, mindfulness provides a steady anchor in life. As meditation teacher Jack Kornfield suggests, it can help you awaken to the 'unshakable freedom'[68] of being fully alive.

REWIRING OUR BRAIN
THROUGH MINDFULNESS

Over the last two decades, research in psychology and neuroscience has shown that the brain's structures are not fixed once we reach adulthood.[69] Rather, our thought patterns and brain structure are adaptable, and we can change and rewire the way our brain works. This idea has been evidenced by studies that have shown how mindfulness leads to neuroplasticity in certain parts of the brain, or the ability for the brain's structure and function to change over time. For psychology these changes have offered a rich new field of study and approach to clinical disorders.

Though studies are still underway and much more research is required, what has interested scientists is tracking the way information moves into our brain through our sensory receptors, or interoceptors. When information comes into the brain, it follows neural pathways that then lead to a thought and/or action. When we repeat thoughts and actions, these neural pathways deepen and become patterns of behaviour. What mindfulness offers is a self-regulatory behavioural process whereby we interrupt the process between the interoceptors firing and following the same neural pathway. By choosing a different route we start to create different responses to situations such as pain, emotional stress or anxiety. This allows us to positively affect our responses.

STARTING A PRACTICE

What is it exactly to be mindful, and what does a mindfulness practice look like? The most common form of practice is seated meditation. You can sit on a cushion or chair, or if you have an injury you can lie down (see Chapter 8, pages 106–7). You can start with the breath-based meditations, which are the entry point for mindfulness. The difference now is to begin working with the thoughts, feelings and sensations that arise. As you become aware of them, notice your response. Do you tighten more? If so, notice the tightening and then gently soothe the tension and return to your breath. Do you feel restless and fidgety? If so, then notice the restlessness and extend care and steadiness towards it, like the way you might help calm an agitated, squirming child.

As mindfulness is about the ability to respond skilfully to situations, it is not restricted to sitting down formally in quiet meditation, though this can serve as a helpful ground to begin developing awareness of the tendencies of our mind. One valuable aspect of mindfulness is that it can be practised in everyday life. In the next section on 'cultivating mindfulness' you can choose ways to focus your practice and develop the skills you need to meet experiences with more presence, spaciousness and gentleness.

The basic idea in mindful practice can be summarised with the Three Cs and Three Rs. The Three Cs were taught to me by my teacher Martin Aylward. They have become a solid framework with which I have learned to practise mindfulness, and continue to be an invaluable resource. They are:

- **CONTACT**: Make contact with something in your body happening now, such as your breath, a sound or sensation. This is the foundation of your practice, and where you can establish and re-establish presence.

- **CURIOSITY**: When you practise, be curious about experience. What is arising? What is felt? Can you track your experiences and pay close attention with interest and enthusiasm? Martin often uses a French phrase to describe this: à l'écoute, which means 'to be on the listen for'. Notice what is happening more and more in your experience.

- **CARE**: As sensations, thoughts and feelings arise, care for them. This is important, as very often you will condemn what arises! You can easily feel you're no good at meditation or mindfulness when you inevitably feel sleepy, fidgety, lost in thought or are somehow harsh on your experience. Extend care instead towards whatever arises. Be gentle in the way you bring awareness back from thinking to something like the contact of your body breathing.

The Three Rs are also a good reference for paying attention and orientating your mindfulness practice. They are:

- **RECOGNISE**: Begin by recognising what is happening. Are you thinking? Worrying? Planning? Fantasising?

- **RELEASE**: When you recognise what is happening, this allows you the opportunity to release it. Softly let go and free up whatever might have lassoed your experience and dragged it away.

- **RETURN**: Come back to something happening in the present moment, such as your breath, sounds or a bodily sensation.

To begin practising mindfulness, start with these two goals:

1. **START A DAILY SITTING PRACTICE:** Begin with 10 minutes a day. Follow a guided meditation. There are many available for free online or via mobile apps (see the additional resources listed at the end of this book). Rather than trying to find time at some point during the day, try to schedule a regular time slot each day. Try not to miss a day. Remember: it's better to sit for a shorter time than to miss a day completely.

2. **PRACTISE BEING MINDFUL IN EVERYDAY LIFE:** Pick an activity you engage in each day to do mindfully. For example, brushing your teeth, washing the dishes, taking a shower, making a cup of coffee, doing your yoga, qigong or other mind–body exercise practices.

CULTIVATING MINDFULNESS

Cultivating mindfulness nurtures the fields of our hearts and minds. It provides you with tools that help sustain and support greater resilience, awareness and the freedom to live a full and enriching life. Here are a few ways.

MINDFULNESS OF BODY

The first aspect of mindfulness taught by the Buddha was mindfulness of the body. The body offers a steady anchor for experience for when you are caught up in thoughts. The sensations and qualities of bodily life provide an actual experience you can use to focus your mind when it wanders, craves, demands or feels stress. By paying attention with kindness towards the physical experience of something – such as your breath or parts of your body – you can learn to shift away from concepts and stories that may seduce your thoughts into direct, immediate experience.

When practising mindfulness of the body, you can learn to develop greater receptivity to the moment-to-moment events that take place in your body. Everything in your experience arises from your body. You may think things only happen in your mind or emotions with no physical correlation, but there is ALWAYS a physical dimension to any mental and emotional state. When you can begin perceiving this more acutely, you can learn skills to deal with situations, such as when tension builds, by learning ways to consciously relax. This awareness of your body can lead to feeling a greater level of receptivity and responsiveness in your life.

Regular practice of mindfulness of body lets you foster deeper respect, care and even wonder and reverence for the body. This is not always easy of course. Many people harbour trauma in the body or narrate stories about how the body should look or feel. I did this for years. As a dancer and then yoga teacher, I started out believing I should conform to a certain stereotyped weight and look. This led to judging and resenting my body in ways that undermined my happiness. With mindfulness of body practices, however, I recognised that while I do not always have to love my body, I can respect and care for it. This began an important shift in letting judgements soften. In time, I was able to see past the form and look into the miracle of neurological sophistication at work just to keep the body alive.

The Buddha described practising mindfulness of the body in six primary ways. This is a summary based on his concepts, put through a contemporary language and framework:

1. **BREATH** – We looked at learning to calm and concentrate the mind by focusing on the breath in Chapter 8. A focus on breath is a common and very immediate way of practising mindfulness of the body (see pages 110–1 for descriptions of mindful breathing).

2. **POSTURE** – This can be sitting, standing, lying down, and something in between. Standing or walking can be a very

quick way to feel embodied, as you learn to pay attention to what moves or keeps you upright.

3. **ACTIVITIES, INCLUDING EATING, DRINKING, GETTING DRESSED, SPEAKING** – These ordinary activities are a rich field for exploring mindfulness. An exercise of mindful eating is described overleaf.

4. **BODY PARTS** – This includes everything in the body, from the feet to the crown and all the parts in between. Practise scanning the body; bringing awareness from the crown of the head to your eyes, mouth, jaw, throat, shoulders and downwards through the whole body can be an excellent way to pay attention to what is here.

5. **ELEMENTS** – These refer to five elements that ancient Indian traditions, such as yoga and Buddhism, believed comprise the human body. These are slightly different to the Chinese Five Elements. In Buddhism and yoga these elements are earth, water, fire, air and ether. With earth you can sense into the stability and density of your body. With water, feelings of fluidity or cohesion. With fire, feelings of heat or coolness. With air, expansion and contraction, such as through the breath. With ether, the spaces in the body, such as the nostrils, ears and mouth. Notice all of these as sensations and experiences within the body that arise and dissolve.

6. **CHANGING EXPERIENCE** – Everything in your body undergoes a process of growth, change and decay. As you practise mindfulness of body, you begin to zero in on this idea and learn to gently accept that this process at work within you is also constantly at work all around you. Knowing this can help you let go of a need for certainty, and become open to the fluid, indefinite nature of all experience.

PRACTICES FOR MINDFULNESS OF BODY

1. **WALKING OR STANDING MEDITATION:** While walking to/from work or any location, or while standing and waiting for a tube or bus, in a queue etc., come fully into direct experience with your physical sensations: notice your arms, legs, feet, hands. Notice when 'narrative/thinking mind' starts and gently bring attention back to your physical sensations.

2. **EATING MEDITATION:** At least once a week, eat part of your meal with full attention to physical sensations. Observe the smell, sight and sound of food; the sensations in your belly; the feel of each bite; swallowing sensations; an urge to prepare the next mouthful before you have finished the first. When you get lost in thought and 'eat mindlessly', gently bring attention back to the sensations of eating.

MINDFULNESS OF FEELINGS – THE PLEASANT, UNPLEASANT AND NEUTRAL

The Buddha describes all phenomena arising in our bodily experience and thoughts as falling into three categories: pleasant, unpleasant or neutral. He called these the *vedana*, which roughly translates as 'feeling tones'. These feeling tones are not feelings as we tend to think of them; they are not feeling sad, happy, hot or cold. Rather, the *vedana* elicit certain reactions in our experience. For example, when something unpleasant happens, such as a loud fire alarm going off in the middle of a yoga class, most people will recoil or cover their ears. If something pleasant happens, such as a friend arriving with a gift, we like this and give them a smile or a hug. Neutral is a bit of a trickier tone to understand. Usually it is present when we are bored or lose interest. I often feel myself slide into neutral when I am calling for telephone support and the operator puts me on hold for fifteen minutes!

Martin Aylward describes these tendencies as the Three Ds, or three primary habits of reacting towards the pleasant, unpleasant and neutral:

1. **DEMANDING** – When we like something and it arouses a pleasant response in us, we lean towards it and demand more from it. You may like the way a glass of wine tastes so you have a second or third glass.

2. **DEFENDING** – When we do not like something and it arouses an unpleasant response, we pull away from it and defend against it.

3. **DISTRACTING** – When something is not very interesting, we move outwards and space out. We become distracted.

These are useful images as they offer a physical movement that you can sense happening when one of these feeling tones is triggered.

Understanding how you respond to pleasant, unpleasant and neutral stimulation is one of the richest grounds of mindfulness practice. When you become aware of your reactive tendencies and give yourself space to pause and respond, you start to see and then free yourself from repeating the same pattern. This is insightful and liberating.

Here are four ways to work with the feeling tones of pleasant, unpleasant and neutral:

1. **UNGRASP.** When something pleasant arises and you begin to cling, simply notice and allow for the pleasantness of the experience without demanding more. Let go and ungrasp.

2. **SOFTEN.** When you meet with the unpleasant, soften your defences. Notice and allow the unpleasantness of the unpleasant. If it's too intense, shift attention away. If it's something small and insignificant, such as your partner not putting away the dishes after a meal, then relax around it

and give yourself space. Work with the 'view of vastness' from Daoism. Remember this is not the only thing happening in the universe. Remember that your current story is not the only story happening in life.

3. **LABEL**. Start to label your experience. Say 'frustrating' when something bothers you. 'Sadness' when something triggers a tear. 'Freaking out' when you feel extremely wound up or overly agitated. Point the way towards the possibility of allowing these feelings space, or the idea of freeing them. This is the process called 'affect labelling', where we put our feelings into words. Studies have shown that this process helps alleviate negative emotional responses by quieting down the amygdala, the part of the brain that processes emotions, decision-making and fear responses.[70]

4. **INVESTIGATE**. Explore what has triggered your reactivity; what has led to the experience you have labelled as pain, or the experiences that upset and wind you up. Pay attention to the present experience, rather than the backstory that can easily seduce you. Make a choice in how you respond to these stimuli instead of habitually reacting or repeating old patterns.

MINDFULNESS OF THOUGHTS

Why would we want to work with our thoughts? Are they something we can even change? The French philosopher René Descartes famously proclaimed, 'I think, therefore I am', so do thoughts not define who we are? The answer to this is yes, we can change our thoughts, and thinking is actually just one aspect of who we are. We are also embodied, feeling organisms.

Working with mindfulness gives you an opportunity to cultivate a wiser relationship with your thoughts and to diminish your tendencies towards undermining self-judgement. We will look at self-judgement in Chapter 11. For now let us look at ways we can understand thoughts and what tools mindfulness can give us to meet them.

Very often we are lost in thought. This leads to feeling separate from what is actually happening in the here and now. You may be at the top of a mountain on a sunny, clear day, but all you can think about is why he did not text you back, should I have written him something different, could I have acted differently? When you are lost in thoughts, it is like living your life on autopilot. You have less control over the direction and orientation of what you choose to do or where you choose to place your energy and attention.

It is estimated that we have between 15,000 and 90,000 thoughts per day. That means that we can have one thought every .48 seconds! Of these thoughts how many will be clear, compassionate, wise and insightful? How many are random or end up creating mental clutter? How many are detrimental, harmful, damaging or corrosive? How many do we habitually react to without even realising? Becoming mindful of your thoughts allows you to reflect on this. When you begin to illuminate your thinking habits, gradually you will begin to see which thoughts are random and harmful, and which are clear, logical and useful. With mindfulness of thinking you can identify which thoughts are not useful and drop them, or slowly work on transforming them into insights. This is the practice of wise discernment.

MINDFULNESS OF THOUGHT EXERCISE: DROP THE BANANA

I once read that in Thailand people catch monkeys using a simple device. They take a coconut, cut a hole in it, place a banana inside, and then secure the coconut by tying a rope to a heavy rock or tree. The monkey will try to reach inside the coconut to take the banana and becomes stuck. It refuses to let go and ends up trapped while still grasping the banana. We are often trapped like this monkey with thoughts and stories that repeat in our heads. We often refuse to drop the banana and get stuck in unskilful thinking. If you can remember that you always have the choice of dropping the thoughts and stories that trap you, you can set yourself free. Practise dropping the banana whenever you can.

MINDFULNESS OF EMOTIONS

When we feel a strong emotion, we often do one of two things: identify with it, or push it away. Identifying with an emotion is built into our language: I feel angry. I am sad. Mindfulness of emotions teaches us that you can follow a different path to meet emotions and work to gradually soften their grip. This helps foster four important qualities:

1. **RESILIENCE**: you expand your capacity to adapt to stressful situations and build greater emotional steadfastness.

2 **NON-ATTACHMENT/DISASSOCIATION**: you learn to separate the story from the direct experience or state of what you feel.

3. **RESPONSIVENESS**: you discern emotions as they arise and detect them earlier and with greater clarity. This enables you the freedom to respond to emotions so that they do not ensnare you in reactivity and cause ongoing suffering.

4. **COMPASSION**: your appreciation for and expressions of greater compassion and kindness. As your awareness and mindfulness of emotions develop, this can foster greater empathy and compassion for others.

Here is a personal story about how working with mindfulness of emotions can be a difficult but rewarding process. A number of years ago during my mindfulness training, I was standing outside doing a nature-based meditation. The wind was blowing lightly, and it caused my hair to start tickling my face. I wanted to pull my hair back or scratch my face, but then I stood still and didn't move, thinking, I can allow this to just be unpleasant and soften around it. But suddenly a memory of when my father was ill in the intensive care unit of the hospital came up. He had been in and out of the ICU and surviving on life support. This was in Taiwan, where doctors often keep patients conscious after being on life support for a number of days. While my father was intubated and on life support, he was often visibly uncomfortable. He could not speak, but would sometimes reach his hands slowly towards his face. I imagined he was trying to scratch an itch, but the nurses thought he was trying to pull out his tube. As a result, the staff decided that anytime the family was not there with him, they would bind and tie his hands down so that he would not try to pull the tube out.

This memory filled me with anger, shame, guilt, and very quickly sadness and grief also came up – I was mourning my father. He had only passed a year ago. I felt the sadness start to overwhelm me. It rose up through me like a heat, and I wanted to do one of three things: 1) start crying and run like hell from the standing meditation; 2) make these feelings and thoughts go away as fast as possible; or 3) go more into the story and think about all the other things that went wrong then. I could have easily been seduced by more and more memories and thoughts that would have kept me in a downwards spiral of even more sadness and grief, maybe even more anger and blame – at myself, the doctors, or anyone I could think of.

Instead, I practised a tool I had learned for mindfulness of emotions called R.A.I.N., which was developed by Michele McDonald. It stands for:

1. **RECOGNISE** (name it/label it),

2. **ALLOW** (accept and not try to fix),

3. **INVESTIGATE** (be curious about how the emotion feels in your BODY with a kind attention: is it in your chest? Solar plexus? Stomach?) and

4. **NOT PERSONAL/NON-IDENTIFICATION** (the emotion does not define you, remembering that 'this too shall pass').

Standing there, I began allowing the sensations to arise. I practised the 'R' of recognise. I saw the sadness, anger, blame and grief boiling up in me. I granted it some space, and then practised the 'I' as I investigated it – where am I feeling these sensations in my body right now? I began to shift away from the memory and story towards asking, 'What is the direct experience of this for me right now?' I started to feel physical sensations in my heart and chest – it felt awful in those places, simultaneously hollow, heavy and like an icy burn. As I met these feelings in my body, I continued to inquire – 'How are they experienced right now?' Then I allowed them to be and recognised their impermanence – they arose from the wind blowing, and just as they arose they could pass. The sadness and grief were there and valid, but I could watch these feelings and thoughts arise and also watch them pass and soften. Within a few minutes I felt lighter, softer, more spacious and more able to breathe. The burning, icy heaviness was gone. I was back in the open air again, with the wind, sun and nature there. Me standing. No more itch, like a tornado had appeared from nowhere and just as swiftly moved on. I stood there resting in a wakeful and open freedom. The story of my father's suffering had passed, and I was no longer gripped by the guilt, shame and anger that surrounded his suffering. I still missed him terribly, but I recognised that this was because I loved him so much. This can be the fruit of R.A.I.N.: new possibility, new growth and flowering.

It's also important to note, however, some emotions may be too strong to meet with R.A.I.N. If this is true, begin with smaller steps. Practise R.A.I.N. when you feel mild irritation or slight hurt, but not debilitating anger or grief. Cultivate your threshold incrementally and meet your emotions gently. Learn to skilfully respond to them. In time, your thoughts and emotions can become transformed into places of learning, compassion and wisdom.

MINDFUL MOVEMENT

Mindfulness can also be developed through movement practices such as yoga, qigong, tai chi or a walk in nature. These practices tend to be slower, focused in the body, and involve a deepening awareness of how and why we move. This is different to walking or running on a treadmill while watching the evening news and trying to forget about the body's exertion and fatigue. Neuroscientists, such as Catherine Kerr, advocate the benefits of mind–body-centred movement on the brain, pointing out the overall positive effects these movement arts have in reducing inflammation (which is a leading cause of heart disease, diabetes and dementia), as well as our ability to regulate emotion.[71]

Qigong and tai chi are unique movement-based practices in the way they use intention to direct our energy flow. In Chinese medicine and qigong there is a saying, 'yi dao qi dao' (意道氣道), which means 'energy goes where intention flows'. For example, you might be instructed to move the hands like clouds, which immediately suggests a softness and ease to the action, or to push mountains with the hands, which calls on more force and strength from the hands as well as from the whole body. For this reason, practices tend to be slower to give practitioners time to visualise these actions. There is also more time for the mind and body to co-ordinate their efforts. The relationship between the body and brain is something researchers in the field of cognitive science and embodied awareness are beginning to study more closely.[72]

In yoga there are many approaches to practice, reflecting different speeds, lineages and goals. When I teach and practise yoga, I integrate ideas from mindfulness to help create a more compassionate relationship to the practice for my students. This means the practice is not just about performing postures, concentrating and sensing the breath (which are all valuable), but also about how we can become more aware of our mental and emotional tendencies as they arise. To help with this I often teach what I have called 'Yoga 3D'. This approach helps students work with their experience and allows them to meet postures with more clarity, awareness and insight.

MINDFULNESS IN YOGA: YOGA 3D – DECELERATE, DE-AGGRAVATE, DISENTANGLE

If you practise yoga, you may know that one of the main benefits can be releasing tension and calming the mind through a combination of physical postures, breathing and meditation. The purpose, process and outcome of yoga is to help you consciously begin to relax into life. It lets you begin to see past the confusion, ignorance, misunderstandings and delusions. When you begin to look beyond these obstacles, you begin to see the truth of what is actually here, which is life happening live. It helps you see things more clearly.

To support this process and allow the practice of yoga postures to become more than just ways to move, stretch and strengthen the body, I developed 'Yoga 3D'.

- **DECELERATE** when you feel like you are going too fast. Slow down if you feel yourself speeding through the practice.

- **DE-AGGRAVATE** when you start to feel like you are annoyed, upset or making a situation worse. Ease out of annoyance if you start to feel frustrated or like you are pushing yourself unnecessarily hard or feeling too aggressive in the practice.

- **DISENTANGLE** from anything unnecessarily complex. Keep things simple and disentangle your thoughts: when your mind wanders away from your downward-facing dog, come back to the breath and the sensations of the body.

Practising Yoga 3D on the mat can also help you move mindfulness from the formal practice into everyday activities. Here is where you can truly witness the fruits of the practice ripen and bring balance to your life.

THE FRUITS OF MINDFULNESS

Though I have been meditating regularly since 2002 and practising yoga since 1995, I did not always approach these practices mindfully. For years I believed I should practise with a specific goal of stilling the fluctuations of my mind. This is what I had been taught was the goal of yoga. This aim had benefits: it taught me how to concentrate and quieten my mind. When I began to shift towards becoming mindful of my thoughts, it was like taking the blinkers off a horse. Suddenly everything was exposed. Paying attention and learning to respond to the avalanche of my thoughts was a revelation. No one ever taught me this in school.

The light bulb that switched on is knowing I can actually do something with my thoughts other than let them ramble or try to block them. This was fascinating, humbling and insightful. Mindfulness helped me see how terrible I was at times in judging or blaming myself, but also how I could open myself up to compassion. It showed me how distracted I usually was, but how I could also come back to something here and present, like my breath. Though I am still sometimes hard on myself and often distracted, I now feel more equipped to deal with these tendencies when they arise. I can cultivate less negativity and judgement and more kindness and caring attention towards my thoughts and emotional states. I can identify which seeds are weeds and which are flowers. I am gradually learning to stay with experience, which helps me feel less fragmented and more in tune and aligned with everything that is all around me.

What I discovered – and I hope you will also experience this as part of your xiu yang practice – is that mindfulness can help you create a wiser relationship with your thoughts and emotions. Through this you begin to open up to greater insight, compassion and freedom – to yourself and the world around you.

10

A Harmonious Heart

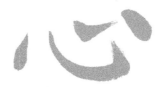

The ancient Chinese believed that the heart's natural capacity was like the midday sun: radiant, warming, spacious and expansive. They believed the heart supports our life and infuses it with qualities that make us complete as human beings.[73] The things that interfere with this process are strong emotions, such as anger, grief, desire and even excessive joy. This is why xiu yang's approach to the heart is so important. It invites us to remember the heart's innate capacity to be free, while cultivating practices that gently smooth out the ways it can feel imbalanced. When our heart's energies are strengthened, restored and realigned, we can begin to see our capacity for health, happiness and balance naturally emerge.

THE HEART HOLDS PARADOX

In the West we tend to think of our hearts and minds as holding distinct roles and responsibilities. The mind is where logical, clear reason takes place, and the heart where our emotional life abides. Emotions, as defined by the Oxford Dictionary, are instinctive and intuitive feelings as distinguished from reasoning or knowledge.[74] In making decisions we often face an either/or dilemma: listen to our head or follow our heart – never both. In this tug of war usually the head wins.

The problem, however, is that our mind dislikes turning grim, ambiguous or uncertain corners. It prefers having logical, clear answers. If someone breaks up with us, we want to know why and what we may have done wrong. When someone close to us dies, we want to know why, how and what could have been done. Our efforts to understand are important and should not be overlooked. But sometimes our need to find answers makes our mind tighten. It also prevents us from opening to the complexity of the whole situation or working with difficult emotions, such as heartache, grief and pain. Break-ups are messy. The sudden death of a loved one never feels fair or easily explained. The heart, however, can meet these situations and hold them. This is because the heart is designed to hold paradox.

In Chinese this ability of the heart to hold paradox makes sense. The heart is known as the *xin* (心), which has an emotional as well as cognitive function. If someone feels sad, it is because their heart is *xin suan* (心酸), which means it is bitter. If someone has a strong capacity for clear thinking, it is because they are very *xin qiao* (心竅), which means their heart is good at finding solutions. The same is true in yoga and Buddhism. In both traditions the *citta* is consciousness, but it can also be translated as the heart, mind or heart-mind. *Xin* is also translated by some as heart-mind, such as in the *Inward Training* chapters I have included in this book.

If you meet uncertain or difficult experience with your heart, your emotions and thoughts do not have to stand at odds but can instead become united and strong. This gives you a far greater ability to respond to life's challenges and difficulties. You can simultaneously feel the heartbreak of what you see in the news while also responding to the sweetness of a child's laugh. When in balance, you can hold life's paradoxes gently by combining the heart's knowing with tenderness and care. When you learn to open to the fuller range of your human heart, you begin to cultivate a stronger, tender and more compassionate approach to life's challenges.

Over the years I have shared the heart's ability to hold paradox with students, and it has helped many create a new perspective on difficult situations such as divorce and break-up. One student, Kim, recently told me that thinking of her ex-husband caused feelings of anger, frustration and impatience to swell up in her. Yet when she moved out of her head and into feeling with her heart, she noticed space for compassion for him, and the ability to be OK with the pain, confusion and sadness of their situation.

Another student, Charli, was going through a hard break-up when I shared this ability of the heart to hold a wide range of experience. Afterwards she posted this insight from our conversation on social media:

> I had a very enlightening chat with my yoga teacher after class yesterday. She said the mind wants answers, logical explanations and rationale. It sees things in black and white. That's where the 'why me?' and 'it's not fair' comes from as well as the overwhelming emotions that follow during a break-up. But the heart is stronger; it can accept duality ... I remember experiencing tears of sadness and laughter with beautiful friends in the very same moment six years ago in India. I was so confused in that moment to what I was feeling. How could I cry and laugh in the same breath? Now I understand how that was possible. I have been using this new skill and it's working. Any time my mind starts thinking and wanting answers I just drop down to my heart, feel the sadness and the happiness at the same time, and know that everything is OK.

Charli's ability to move out of her mind and into the terrain of her heart was a tender example of meeting experience through the courage and capacity of her heart. Her willingness to recognise heartache as running parallel to beauty unfolding around her allowed her to heal more quickly.

CULTIVATING THE HEART

Meditation and mindfulness are practices that awaken the heart to our full human incarnation, with its immense suffering and unimaginable beauty. This is because the practices help you cultivate a heart that is less captivated by compulsions, fears and anxieties and more inclined towards compassion, love and kindness. In the midst of a celebration you open to joy fully. When you face sadness and loss, you summon the strength, compassion and care to help you move through it with the least harm to yourself or others while also giving love and support to those who are in pain. In time you can proficiently use tools that help you cultivate a heart that is freer and brighter like the sun. This helps align the heart, which in Chinese is called *zheng xin* (正心), and move towards an integrated sense of wholeness, known as *cheng yi* (城意). In *Inward Training* this process also allows us to touch into the Dao itself:

> *The Dao is without a set place;*
> *But the calmness of an adept heart-mind makes a place.*
> *When the heart-mind is still and qi is patterned,*
> *The Dao may come to rest.*
> *Such a way is not remote from us –*
> *When people realise it, they are thereby sustained.*
> *Such a way is not separate from us –*
> *When people accord with it, they are thereby harmonious.*

Inward Training (Neiye), Chapter 5[75]

Here are three meditation and mindfulness practices that specifically can help you cultivate a harmonious heart. They are a combination of physical movements, visualisations and meditations.

XIU YANG FOR SOFT HANDS

The hands are believed to be messengers of the heart. In Chinese medicine the meridian lines for the heart and its helpers run from the fingers through the hands, arms and into the torso. In psychology handshakes communicate certain inclinations: a limp hold can be perceived as lacking interest in the person you are greeting, while a firm, bone-crushing grip conveys dominance.[76]

The hands are also hard-wired to our brain. There are numerous motor skills required to enable our hands to gesticulate, grasp and create, which generates a considerable amount of neurological traffic between our hands and brains. You also have some of the densest areas of nerve endings in your fingers, which makes them sensitive and tactile. This could have been one reason why in nineteenth-century Europe women were prescribed knitting as an activity to calm anxiety. New research by Kelly Lampert, a neuroscientist at the University of Richmond, suggests that when we do something with our hands we also calm the brain and can change its neurochemistry; making something with your hands, such as cooking, painting or putting things together, can calm and engage the brain in positive ways.[77]

These two exercises that follow are aimed at helping you soften your hands, quiet the mind and calm the heart. You can do any of these practices on their own or combine them into a ten-minute meditation on relaxing the hands.

CLOUD HANDS/
MOVING HANDS LIKE CLOUDS

This is a practice from qigong and tai chi. In this exercise visualise your hands becoming soft yet strong agents that are capable of moving delicate pillow-like clouds. Do this in a way that is as natural and effortless as possible. Keep your breathing natural, steady and relaxed.

1. Stand with your feet hip distance apart. Bend the knees slightly. Relax the joints of the body. Now bring your hands towards your centre, right hand above the left, palms facing

each other. Keep the hands separated by 30–40 cm (12–15 inches). Imagine the hands are holding clouds.

2. Begin to move the clouds between your hands towards the right, turning your waist gently. As you move the imaginary clouds, keep the lower hand at the level of your lower abdomen, and the top hand just below your ribs on the mid-chest.

3. Once you turn to a comfortable degree, switch the position of your hands by rolling your right hand down as you bring the left hand above, palms facing again. Then move the hands smoothly towards the left, turning your waist gently.

4. Continue and repeat, moving the hands from side to side slowly and calmly. Imagine your hands move like water in a stream – fluid, unbroken and steady.

5. When you finish, bring the hands back in towards your centre and turn them so that the palms face each other with the thumbs pointing towards the sky. Gently release the hands, palms facing down, releasing the clouds that you moved between them.

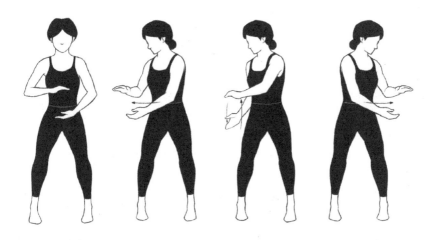

RECLINING BUDDHA

This is a meditation with a simple focus: relaxing your hands as thoroughly as you can while lying on your side. When I did my yoga teacher training with Erich Schiffmann, he assigned this one day as homework. He called this form the 'Reclining Buddha', named after the position the Buddha chose to take as he entered into Nirvana and ended all his reincarnations. The posture is known as *shiasaiyas*, the posture of a sleeping or reclining lion.

Lie down on your right side, bend the knees, and reach your right arm overhead. Prop your head on to your arm. Place your left hand on the top hip. Relax it as much as you can. Then relax it even more. Continue relaxing your hand until it feels like melted butter. Stay with this feeling for a few minutes, then slowly change sides and repeat on the other side. Finish by rolling on to your back and resting one hand on your belly and one hand on your heart. It does not matter which hand goes where. Simply notice the hands relaxing and breathe deeply.

METTĀ: THE PRACTICE OF CARE

This practice is a meditation on *mettā*, which involves cultivating care and happiness from the heart towards ourselves and others. *Mettā* is often translated into English as 'loving-kindness'. I often think that if I'd told my father, an engineer and scientist, that he should practise more loving-kindness, he would probably have met my request with scepticism, and perhaps even stopped listening to what I had to say. This is because things he considered new-age jargon usually put him off. If I'd suggested that he practise more care, however, he might have been compelled to try. I therefore prefer the translation of *mettā* as 'care', which is what our heart needs the most when it aches.

The practice of *mettā* may be challenging to some. Especially if you are feeling low, turning care towards yourself or others may not be your first inclination. Yet this recognition itself is part of mindfulness training: when you become present and aware of your habit to push away care for yourself, notice it and become aware of what it triggers in you. Make a choice to meet your feelings gently. Gently make some space for the pushing away, which can soften your resistance to it. In soothing the difficulty you may experience an opening to allow for some care to be extended towards yourself. This is why *mettā* is a practice of mindfulness: it reminds you that you can choose to respond with wisdom and insight towards obstacles and struggle.

It should also be noted that while regular *mettā* practice can open us to step into rich and rewarding territory, many of us may have a hard time extending care towards ourselves. This is because our conditioned tendencies are difficult to change. It can be far easier to take care of and extend love to others – partners, friends, pets or plants – and difficult to extend love and care to oneself. Being willing to work gently with the heart and offer practices to support its optimal function, however, can begin to bring forth the heart's inherent capacity to give and receive love. This is tremendously healing.

Within the mindfulness tradition there are specific meditations on *mettā*. While most *mettā* meditations begin with a focus on extending *mettā* to oneself, I prefer to begin *mettā* with a focus on someone easy to love. In part, extending love to another person feels more natural to me, and may also offer you an effective strategy for working around awkward feelings that can arise when practising acts of self-love. Extending love to another person creates an opening in the heart. This allows you to more easily give care to yourself.

1. Sit quietly on a cushion or chair and begin to sense into your own heart. Take a few moments to send soft breath into the area of your heart. Place your hands on your energetic heart centre, which is the centre of your chest.

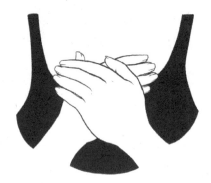

2. Bring to mind someone easy to love, and whose relationship with you is uncomplicated. This can be a child, pet, nephew or niece. Allow time for the person's (or animal's) image to form in your mind and feel their presence nearby. Then begin to repeat these words silently to yourself:

'May they be happy. May they be healthy and well.
May they be safe and protected. May they be at ease and feel peace'.

3. Repeat these phrases three to five times.

4. Focus your attention on yourself, and your own heart. Take a few breaths to let this attention feel sincere, generous and kind. When you feel ready, repeat these words to yourself:

'May I be happy. May I be healthy and well.
May I be safe and protected. May I be at ease and feel peace'.

5. Repeat these phrases three to five times.

6. Extend the practice out to others in your life. Start with someone neutral, like your postman. Then extend *mettā* to someone difficult in your life. Finish by extending *mettā* to all beings. Repeat the words, 'May they be happy. May they be healthy and well. May they be safe and protected. May they be at ease and feel peace.' Repeat these phrases three to five times.

7. Finish by sensing into your heart. What is the quality present for you?

REMEMBERING YOUR
HEART'S INNATE GOODNESS

Like the soaring and radiant sun, remember that the true nature of the heart is to give effulgent brightness, warmth, steadiness and love. If in doubt of this capacity, step outside and turn your face towards the sun. Even if it is behind clouds, remember that the sun is still there generating the light we are given each day. As T. S. Eliot wrote, 'When the black cloud carries away the sun ... still there is light at the still point of the turning world.'[78] Remembering the light of the sun can be an immediate way to practise xiu yang: cultivating a more harmonious heart by connecting to the source of light that is the sun in our sky.

11

Freeing the Inner Critic:
From Self-Concern
to Self-Cultivation

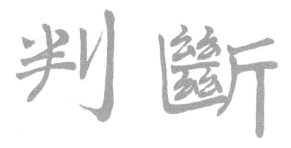

While there are ways to cultivate your heart to feel more aligned and capable of holding life's paradox and ambiguity, sometimes thoughts can be so damaging and cruel that meeting them with gentleness and awareness is not enough. Indeed, when unchecked, certain thoughts can undermine mental and emotional balance, bite into self-worth, and deeply wound your capacity for well-being and joy. These types of destructive thoughts most often come in the form of the inner critic. Critical, damning and judgemental thoughts are like parasitic plants that latch on to a host, debilitate it and gradually suck out its nutrients. The practice of xiu yang can help you identify the nature and presence of these leeching plants and cut them back before they jeopardise your long-term happiness.

What is the inner critic? It is the voice of the judge, tyrant, taskmaster, killjoy, sergeant major, superego, bully and fun-destroyer. It is the voice that tells us we need approval, to be 'seen' or to achieve an impossible standard of perfection. When it takes over, it becomes like a strangle-weed that can weaken and spread disease, making us feel collapsed, ashamed and unworthy. Mark Coleman, author of *Make Peace with Your Mind*, describes how the inner critic has become one of the most significant causes of depression, anxiety and suicide prevalent today.[79] Left to its own devices it becomes a tenacious threat to the core of our being. In its extreme forms it tells us that it is not OK to be who we are, to be human, to be safe.

By including this chapter in *Xiu Yang* my aim is to share some of the ways we can prevent the inner critic from festering into a crippling force. By seeing through the way the inner critic sabotages our minds we gain freedom from the tyranny of this destructive way of thinking. The main way we do this is by making a conscious turn away from relentless stories of 'what is wrong with me?' towards asking: 'how can I cultivate a more generous and accepting attitude towards myself?' This movement can also be understood as a shift from self-concern to self-cultivation. We learn to distinguish between what is healthy discernment – e.g. a constructive need for change – and what is a corrosive and unhelpful pattern of thought.

Importantly, when you begin to do this work, you cannot be immediately cured of the cruelty of your inner critic's voice. This is an ongoing process of xiu yang: a patient tending to the inner field of your heart and mind that helps you grow an outer happiness, harmony and balance.

THE NEGATIVITY BIAS

One of the challenges we face in our attempts to cultivate mental and emotional balance is our proclivity towards negative thinking. We tend to see the negative far more readily than the positive! This is partly due to our brain chemistry. When something happens, our brains react more to stimuli it deems negative. Research has tested this, showing a greater surge in electrical activity in our brains with negative images and stories than positive ones.[80] Psychology calls this tendency the 'negativity bias'. This tendency demonstrates our brain is actually hard-wired to respond more strongly to doom and disaster than it is to good news.

This is useful for paying attention to potential threats. As a species, we have learned to survive largely because we have excelled at dodging danger. The *Homo sapiens* brain is 315,000 years old. Agriculture only began approximately 12,000 years ago, so for around 96 per cent of our time as a species we've lived as hunter-gatherers. With food and shelter often uncertain, and threats from sabre-toothed tigers or other predators, our fears were understandably fanned. But these particular threats no longer exist, and what we need to survive in the modern world is quite different. Life expectancy has increased, innovation has improved our living standards, and the majority of people who live in developed countries have shelter and sufficient (or even surplus) amounts of food to eat. Still, our brains continue to be hyper-vigilant in reacting to perceived threats and fears. More and more these threats stem from stress, pressure or anxiety from our work, family and relationships.

Think back to a time when your negativity bias may have reared its head, perhaps it was during a break-up, challenging job interview, awkward first date or public performance. What was it like? After the experience, did negative thoughts dominate? How long did you dwell on things? How difficult was it to silence biting commentary or harsh self-evaluations? Left unchecked, our brains can easily send us into a tailspin of doubt, anxiety and worry.

The next time you find yourself triggered by your negativity bias, try this: label it as the bias coming up in your head, and consider whether some of your stresses and fears are remnants of your 315,000-year-old brain. The moment you start to see your inclinations, you initiate a positive shift from self-concern to self-cultivation. This will be an effective means of starting to shake the parasitic inner critic off your back.

WHERE DOES OUR INNER CRITIC COME FROM?

Making this shift requires understanding the origins and roots of the critic when it grows out of control. When you ask where the harmful effects of judgement may have started and whether they are actually true, you also begin to cultivate new perspectives on how your sense of self has been shaped and can be reshaped. In many ways this study can become one of the most undervalued practices of xiu yang: the humble process of inquiry.

Education or other authority

Many of us have at some point in our life felt like we were underperforming. Our teacher, parent or sibling may have said things to us along the lines of 'Don't be stupid', 'That's so easy' or 'If you can't do it, then I'll do it'. These types of casual assertions and accusations can easily seep into our conscious or subconscious identity and affect how we see ourselves. Being the youngest of four children and the only girl I have grown up with versions of this narrative. I constantly felt like I needed to catch up with my brothers, who I always felt were smarter, more articulate and more capable than I was.

When someone says something to us that feels hurtful, these are usually words that were never intended to stick. People say things without thinking them through properly all the time. But we might hear these words and absorb their full weight. To combat this we must recognise that these words are simply opinions and views. They are NOT truths. When you understand this, you can learn to challenge the veracity of these ideas. You can also trust that you are no longer that young child and can therefore start to free yourself from the belief that you are not measuring up to someone else's ideal.

As children and adults, we can feel the need for approval from the people we love or even authority figures. Being 'seen' by them validates us. These needs are reinforced at an early age. Children will often proudly show their parents drawings or achievements they have done, saying, 'Look what I did!' Usually, we are happy when we hear a response such as, 'Oh, how beautiful!' or, 'I am so proud of you.' If our parents do not give us the reaction we expect or hope for, we can feel diminished or as though we have somehow fallen short when we do not receive praise. We can also feel overly validated when we receive excessive praise, which leads to problems of the opposite sort: having an aggrandised sense of self. These exchanges often shape how our inner critic matures into adulthood but it can also be assuaged through the skills of learning to silence it through xiu yang.

Cultural and familial conditioning

Personal views and opinions are also shaped by cultural beliefs and familial conditioning, most of which, growing up, we assume to be correct. This is because cultural norms are seen as necessary for inclusion and survival. When we conform to society's expectations, we fit in and begin to follow the creed that we believe will cast a compelling narrative for success.

In America, for example, there is a general culture of expecting people to pull themselves up by their own bootstraps. This feeds a fierce individualism and a need for independence. Working and saving up to buy your first car, being treated equally, and the right to freely express one's individual views are some of the hallmarks of core American values. In China, however, the opposite is true: leveraging connections is the best way to succeed, and in general one's individual opinion and identity are never more important than the collective family good. Typically, Chinese parents try to make their children humble by pointing out all their faults: you're stupid, too fat, too skinny, not filial enough, not rich enough. It can be easy to believe these ideas if you hear them your whole life. Shaming children with guilt about the way they treat parents is another approach. Many parents, for example, will expect to live with their children when they retire, and often will complain that their children are selfish if they do not buy a big enough house to accommodate them.

Fortunately, my parents never laid on too much negative reinforcement or too much guilt, though they did place a lot of pressure on us to do well. They demanded that we excel in school, work hard and respect our elders. In this sense they were typically Confucian. My father did not make it easy for us either; by the time he was thirty-two he had two master's degrees and a PhD in engineering from some of America's top universities. As a result, my brothers and I all strove to try to measure up to certain standards that we invariably felt we missed.

For over a decade, I suspected that my parents felt ashamed that I became a yoga teacher instead of pursuing my career in photojournalism. This was reinforced by the fact that after I had quit photography for some time, my parents continued to introduce me to their friends as a journalist, leaving out the fact that I taught yoga. This feeling of letting down my parents stayed with me until my father's last trip to London. By then he was already weaker from a heart condition, which meant that we mostly relaxed at my home. During his visit, he saw me living my everyday life. Towards the end of the trip, he said to me, 'Mimi, I never knew that when you decided to teach yoga it would change you so much.' Immediately, my brain started firing all the negativity bias alerts: was he going to criticise me? Would he express more disapproval? He then smiled gently, touched my face and said, 'I can see that you are happy, really happy.' In that instant my brain relaxed, my heart softened, and I felt my father's full and complete love. All he wanted was for me to be happy; he did not care that I was no longer a globe-trotting photographer. With his approval the loud voice telling me that I was unworthy of my parents' respect suddenly vanished.

I was fortunate to have my father share this with me, but even his love and kind words did not fully combat the onslaught of the inner critic's voices that had been steering me towards a need for approval and affection from others. What this did allow me to see, however, is that the cultural and familial origins of our beliefs are not necessarily truths. This perspective was liberating. Views are part of conditioning, often deeply rooted and well formed, but also open to investigation, inquiry and curiosity. When you can start to challenge the validity of your critic's voice and understand its origins, you can learn ways to counter the cunningly stealthy way it undermines your happiness.

HEARING THE CRITIC'S VOICE

Once we know the origin of our critic, we can begin to listen for when it arises. This can be difficult, as it is sometimes hard to distinguish between a healthy judgement that points us towards positive change and the vicious, undercutting voice of the critic. Positive judgement may come in the form of recognising that you have gained a bit of weight after a holiday and deciding afterwards to cut back on sweets and do a bit more exercise. If the inner critic hijacks this well-intentioned process, then you begin to hear the incessant snips of your critic telling you, 'You always do this', 'You should have restrained yourself more', 'Now look at how fat you are, and how much work it's going to take to lose this weight', 'You'll never lose this again', etc. These are things we would never say to our friends!

The inner critic can also be quick to judge others. The reasons for judgement can vary, but often it is because what we see is a mirror to our own experience; we are triggered by something in them that we dislike about ourselves. Sometimes judgements can be helpful and make us recognise that we dislike a person for good reasons. If they pose a physical or emotional threat to us, it would be best to keep contact with them to a minimum. Other times, our judgements manifest in nagging at those we love, which can erode a relationship. When you notice yourself judging others, have an open mind about who it is and why you're judging them. Dissect the judgement and look into it more deeply. What precipitated it? Is it about them or about yourself? How does the judgement feel? Do you feel more open or more contracted when you judge another? Usually, unhelpful judgement feels tight, both when directed towards ourselves as well as towards others, whereas helpful judgements can make us feel clearer, and lead to decisions that give us more freedom and ease.

Learning to be mindful of and examining the judgements you have every day can transform into a lifelong practice for self-cultivation. Having clarity around your judgements develops discernment and leads to wisdom, insight and greater compassion for the way you see difficulty, whether that be in your own experience or in the experiences of others. It can also stem the tide of negativity and retrain your brain to not always default to its negativity bias.

STRATEGIES FOR BANISHING THE INNER CRITIC

Here are three strategies that I have found to be very effective in uprooting the underhanded voice of the inner critic.

1. **STOP. THEN INVOKE YOUR PROTECTOR.** Stopping is as simple and difficult as it sounds! Judgement is a form of the inner critic that is insidious and difficult to uproot. It never works to try to reason or argue with the harsh and unforgiving voice of judgement because 1) it always sees itself as right, and 2) it always has to win an argument. The most effective method for meeting judgement is to be firm and authoritative, and then invoke a protector! A protector is a strong figure, such as the wizard Gandalf from *The Lord of the Rings*, who wards off the beast Balrog with his staff, saying, 'YOU SHALL NOT PASS!' My protector is my father. Tibetan Buddhists use protectors to shield them from the harmful attacks of Māra, the demon of greed, hatred, delusion, desire and doubt. To fend off Māra, they invoke the presence of fierce demigods, such as Mahakala, whose fangs and sharp sword are used to cut through judgement and other negative habits of the mind, eventually turning them into compassion. When

you invoke your protector, imagine them standing in front of you, fending off the inner critic with intense power and strength. Then multiply this protector until they surround you in a tight circle. Sit inside the circle, safe and protected from the threat of your inner critic.

2. **USE HUMOUR.** If you took a step back objectively and imagined someone saying things such as 'It is your fault', 'You did this to yourself' or 'You deserved this' to another person, you might see how ridiculous or silly these accusations and harmful ideas would sound. You could also imagine you are saying these accusations to someone you love or care about, such as a good friend or child, or imagine them saying these things to themselves.

3. **TOUCH THE EARTH AND SAY, 'I BELONG HERE.'** For the Buddha the inner critic came in the form of Māra. Māra approached the Buddha on the night before his final awakening and claimed that only he had the right to ultimate awakening, which meant the Buddha's efforts were misleading and false. In the face of this the Buddha – though advanced in his meditation and practice but still a human being like us all – was not completely equanimous, for doubt is hard to shake. He did, however, find a way to overcome the threat from Māra and finally awaken. In the face of doubt the Buddha reached down with his right hand, touched the earth and asked it to bear witness, which it did. The Buddha then said, 'I belong here.' In his gesture the Buddha offered two powerful ideas:

- As much as we may feel unworthy or insecure about our right to be here, we are part of this earth and belong to it as much as the trees, rivers and mountains.

- We sometimes need to call on some back-up resources and connect to forces greater than ourselves. This is one of the most immediate and powerful ways to feel whole and part of the natural world.

THE JUDGEMENT DIARY

One very effective way to begin countering the critic is to make a daily journal of all the times you have judged yourself or judged others. You may be surprised at how frequently judgement sneaks in. It may be while looking in the mirror that you critique your face, body or health, or it may be that you judge someone for the slowness with which they advance in their place at the queue for coffee. You can then ask yourself these questions:

1. Do these judgements contribute to my practice and overall happiness?

2. Does this make me feel more connected to nature or more separate?

3. If it is a judgement towards yourself, ask: how would I feel hearing this from a close friend? And would they ever dare say this to you or ever think something like that about you?

4. If it is a judgement towards others, how would it feel being on the receiving end?

In time you can realise that judgements are just thoughts that you choose to give attention and authority. If it were the voice of a friend telling you these things, you most likely would not tolerate them nagging and speaking so negatively about you for more than a few minutes.

REMEMBERING YOUR ESSENTIAL NATURE

When you feel like you want to withdraw, collapse or you feel rubbish about yourself, always remember that nature is an immediate, available resource that can steady and support you through life. Hearing the sound of birds, feeling the wind or sensing your feet on the earth can remind you of the miracle of simply being and belonging here. There is no fruit that does not ripen or seed that does not grow when the right conditions are present. But because humans have been given consciousness and an ego, we can end up divided and feeling separate from the Dao. An unchecked ego can interfere with our processes of being and becoming, and stand in the way of living with harmony and ease. This is why mindfulness and countering the inner critic are so important: they point you towards the possibility of slowing the momentum of your ego and finding ease once more through knowing your essential nature, which inherently has a right to belong in this world as a happy, healthy and radiant human being.

PART 4

Xiu Yang for a Happier Place in the World

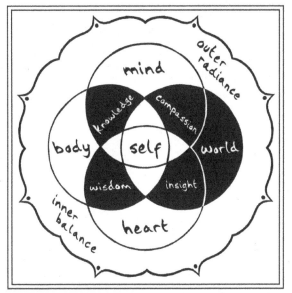

mandala of xiu yang — self-cultivation

Happiness is a universal human desire. In America the Declaration of Independence tells that every person has an inalienable right to 'Life, Liberty and the pursuit of Happiness'. The fourteenth Dalai Lama believes that 'the very purpose of life is to seek happiness'.[81] Living a long and happy life has also always been one of the primary goals in China; xiu yang was the means to achieve this.

What does it mean to be happy? Much of contemporary life – whether that be in Shanghai, Seattle or the south of France – tells us that happiness is feeling accomplishment, a buzz or sudden elation. We are happy when we go on holiday after working day and night to meet a deadline. Our wedding day is often supposed to be the happiest day of our lives. When we are very happy, we say things like 'I am on cloud nine', 'I'm on top of the world' or 'I'm over the moon'. This is because the root word for happy, *hap*, means luck, fortune or chance. Happiness is something temporary and not necessarily a constant state. It is something we earn or are given by chance rather than something we are.

In contrast, the practitioners of xiu yang saw happiness as an inherent, natural state that manifested when one was in harmony with the Dao. Happiness resulted from an internal quality of deep, peaceful calm known as *jing* (靜). This idea of happiness was also shared by ancient Indian and Buddhist teachings, which define happiness as *sukha*. *Sukha* is the opposite of the concept of *dukkha*, which means suffering. Originally, the word *dukkha* referred to an axle that did not fully fit or align with the wheel of an ox cart, which meant a bumpy ride. Suffering is therefore anything in life that makes us squirm, uncomfortable or want things to be different to how they are. In contrast, *sukha* is characterised by a gentle, soothing sense of well-being arising from cultivating meditative states of awareness. There is nothing euphoric about *sukha*. It is not rapture. There are no material attachments or external measures of success associated with it. With *sukha* and *jing* we are shown that happiness is more than a momentary blip on the radar of our lives; it is a consistent point on a tracking system telling us where and how to navigate back to a clear, safe, kind place when life's choppy waters threaten to lose us out to sea.

I remember once reading in a book by Ram Dass a pertinent question: 'Have you ever noticed how many angry people there are at peace rallies?'[82] Rather than meet injustice with anger, xiu yang helps us direct our energy and resources towards an inner harmony and peace that can begin to flourish in the outer world with *sukha* – even when that world is rife with sadness and pain. We are within as we are without. In the words of the poet David Whyte: 'when your eyes are tired, the world is tired also'.[83] Conversely, when we are peaceful, healthy and balanced, the world unfolds in an easier and relaxed way.

Importantly, xiu yang is the path towards these possibilities. By turning towards self-cultivation we can begin to lay important groundwork to meet the world in ways that feel less fraught with incongruity and friction and more open to creating positive change. Without the consistent, intentional encouragement to grow what is healthy and nurturing to ourselves, the qualities of compassion, insight and wisdom can slip through our hands. The trick is remembering that we always need to nurture the right soil. This can take years, but once balanced a good soil naturally grows whatever we plant – including the ability to meet the world in a way that is happier, more open and trusting of life. The Buddha knew this, and current psychological research agrees:[84] our happiness is not fixed but must be consciously cultivated. As we journey into the territory of the world on our mandala of xin yang, we will see how the cultivation of happiness can be best undertaken.

12

Cultivating Virtues for
Sustainable Happiness

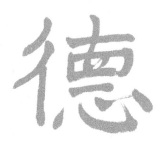

The key concept common to all Chinese philosophy that led to enduring happiness is virtue (*de* 德). In classical Chinese beliefs virtue was a positive agent in life. It was the central path through which a person gained the ability and power to follow their own nature (Dao), and achieve their inherent purpose in life. Ancient Chinese philosophers believed virtue could be applied to a wide spectrum of life, from being humane to pursuing a good education, taking good care of your parents and worshipping one's ancestors. While these ideas remain important in much of Chinese culture today, I will focus on three primary virtues that translate more directly and accessibly and across different times, traditions and cultures.

REN (仁):
HUMANENESS

In Chinese there is a word called *ren* (仁). *Ren* loosely translates into English as 'humane'. In English to be humane means to be tender, fair and kind. Many may see these qualities as positive, but we can also see them in a different way: someone who is tender may be seen as a pushover or too emotional. In a recent conversation with some friends of mine who are economics professors, they said that to succeed in their field they have often been told to develop a thick skin to withstand the intense criticism of their research and work. They also said that they cannot be seen as too invested or sensitive towards their students or colleagues, let alone tender or kind. I, too, remember being told this when I worked in China trying unsuccessfully to run a start-up magazine. Aside from a lack of experience in doing business in China generally, my shortcoming was trying to be too accommodating and fair-minded. In the climate of China's intense race towards capitalism, where many fair business practices and ethics have sadly been cast aside, my attitude flopped.

In classical Chinese thinking *ren* actually refers to more than just being humane. It describes a fundamental ability to be human, love others and create positive interactions.[85] It is the virtue at the root of self-cultivation. This idea was first conceived of by Confucius, who believed rulers should be like sages: wise, knowledgeable, courageous and humane. When *ren* is cultivated within a leader, these virtues naturally radiate outwards and bring universal benefits to all in their domain.[86] In Confucius's words: 'The practice of governance depends on people. One selects people on the basis of one's person; one cultivates one's person according to the Way; and one cultivates the Way according to humaneness.'[87]

To be a leader who is strong and courageous and capable of supporting fair actions guided by wisdom, a person must possess *ren*. They should be a person whose virtues arise from acting authentically and in harmony with the Dao, an inherently benign power and force. Or, as *Inward Training* advised:

> *Govern the heart-mind residing at the centre.*
> *Govern the speech issuing from your mouth*
> *Govern affairs so that they benefit human beings.*
> *Then all under the heavens will be governed.*
> *When the whole meaning is realised,*
> *Then all under the heavens will be covered.*
> *When the whole meaning is stabilised,*
> *Then all under the heavens will be heard.*

Inward Training (Neiye), Chapter 10 [88]

THE IMPORTANCE OF LISTENING

How can you cultivate this quality of humaneness within yourself? In some ways it naturally arises with practices that harmonise and strengthen your body and balance your heart and mind. There are also other things you can do to support your capacity for *ren*. A good starting point is learning how to truly listen to others. This is far more difficult than you might imagine, but in time true listening becomes an incredibly rewarding and enriching practice.

I've always found listening difficult. I grew up in a noisy family where everyone had an opinion, and everyone competed not only to have their opinions heard but to win arguments. Especially among my three older brothers, there was a common belief that if you did not assert yourself quickly, you would be shut out and disregarded. This meant often planning a logical, airtight comeback in the middle of someone else's sentence and rarely actually listening to whoever's opinions were being expressed.

For years I brought this bad habit into the way I communicated. Over time I have learned that by showing others I am listening deeply to what they say, they also soften and listen to me in a more authentic way. By listening first and then trying to understand what someone is communicating we keep a more open mind and less biased view. This helps us remain fair in our judgements and become more attuned to the experience of others. In the yoga teacher training programmes and immersions I lead, I offer practices to the trainees on the art of mindful listening, where one person speaks for between five and ten minutes while the other person simply listens without verbally responding. After these exercises, people often observe how liberating it is to have the space to speak without another person cutting in and offering their advice or opinions.

The most valuable application I have discovered for cultivating mindful listening is in my marriage. It can be easy to make assumptions about what another person thinks or believes, especially when that person is your partner and you assume you know this person well. When you take the time to really listen and forego your opinions and views, you may see that beneath any judgement, blame or hurt is the desire of your partner to be loved and appreciated. Cultivating the ability to listen to them speak without interrupting or becoming argumentative is a way of honouring and respecting their opinions and views. This builds positive communication and deepens respect for the other person. Both of these qualities build a solid foundation for love, which is fundamental to the virtue of *ren*.

When you listen deeply, you see beneath the surface of our experience. In Chinese the character for listening, *ting*, suggests it is more than just hearing someone's words.

聽

In the character for *ting* there are the radicals, or drawings that combine to form words, for the ear but also the heart, the eye and undivided attention. When you listen, you therefore do far more than decipher what someone says. You become present and open your heart to understand deeper meaning. When you listen with sincerity, you cease the constant chatter and tendency to fill a void with radio, television or conversation. Listening requires the support of silence.

CULTIVATING *REN* THROUGH LISTENING

IN NATURE: to listen you must first learn the power of silence. The easiest way to do this is to go out into nature. Take a walk by yourself. Don't take headphones. In fact, leave your phone behind. Embrace solitude. Look down and see how objects in nature, such as grass, shrubs and trees, root silently into the earth. Look up and witness how clouds pass silently in the sky. Take time to listen to the ability of nature to express itself in silence.

IN CONVERSATION: the next time you are in a conversation with someone, feel into your body and sense into the sensations that may be present in your chest or belly. Listen with not just your ears and brain but with your eyes, your heart and your undivided attention. Breathe deeply. Resist the temptation to respond immediately or try to shape opinions about what they are saying and how you will reply. Wait until the person has finished speaking, and then acknowledge what they have said by saying something like, 'It sounds as if you're saying ...' Continue your conversation like this, offering space for them to speak and the intention of understanding them. As you listen, keep your heart open, even if what they say causes friction in your mind. Only when they have finished speaking, offer a response. Let this response come less from your analytical, rational mind and more from your heart.

HUI (惠):
GENEROSITY AND KIND-HEARTEDNESS

Generosity is another virtue that has been cultivated in China for centuries. The classical Chinese understanding of this is *hui*. *Hui* combines the qualities of being giving and kind-hearted. The Buddha emphasised the importance of generosity in his teachings, which is known as *dāna*. *Dāna* is the act of offering things, such as time, money or other resources, freely. It is seen as the first step in the path to awakening because it establishes the foundation for cultivating an open and generous heart. When we give something away without asking for anything in return, such as donating to a charity in times of need, volunteering our time at a school or shelter, or giving alms to a place of worship, we loosen the knots of our attachments that prevent us from awakening to our true Buddha-like nature of freedom and goodness.

In Chinese the notion of generosity is fundamentally linked to the quality of heart, or *xin* (心) (see Chapter 10). One of the reasons I love studying the structure of Chinese characters is because they often join different ideas together in beautiful imagery. The character for *hui* has *xin* as its base. The top of the character originally meant chariot, though today it also means car (車).

We can therefore interpret *hui* as taking the chariot of our heart and riding the gifts of generosity and kind-heartedness into the world.

The act of giving freely brings us a natural joy at every stage. When you think about giving a gift to someone you care deeply about, you think of the person, what they might like, the excitement around what they will think of it, and how it might bring them pleasure and make them feel appreciated and loved. One of my best friends, Mayling, who unfortunately died suddenly at the age of forty-four, was one of the best gift-givers I knew. She put special thought and consideration into the gifts she gave, and never did she expect the same in return. Her knack of giving special gifts was also reflected in a generosity of spirit; she always made time for people, and often went out of her way to help colleagues, students (she was a university professor) and friends. The Buddha's teachings tell us that when people are generous, others love them.[89] This was certainly true of Mayling. One friend described her as 'the antidote to cynicism'. She was a naturally joyous, happy person who was loved and adored by many.

While giving freely to others begins to awaken a sense of inner brightness and joy, the other side of generosity and kind-heartedness is making sure you give equally to yourself. Giving to yourself does not have to be seen as narcissistic or selfish. Attending to your own experiences helps you continue to give to others. From a biological perspective your heart naturally does this: it feeds itself the most oxygen-rich supply of blood first before circulating it to the body's other organs. In the years of teaching yoga, qigong and meditation I have taken this example of the heart and applied it to myself in my role as a teacher. My daily practice is non-negotiable. Every morning I set aside time to cultivate my body, mind and heart. Ideally, I take two hours, though on some days it is as little as a few minutes to simply sit, breathe and attend to what's here. Without this time each day I would not be able to be of service to my students without depleting myself. For my dear friend Mayling I often wonder whether she gave so much to others that there was little left for herself. Though she died peacefully in her sleep, her death was caused by heart complications, which many of her closest friends and family had not realised were as serious as they were. We all wish she had reached out to us to help her carry her burdens, which included increased pressure from work and illness in her family, and let us do what we could to give to her our love, support and care.

Generosity grows and feeds abundance. It is a feeling that we have enough within ourselves to share with others. This sense of abundance is not dependent on income or wealth. Some of the richest people in the world may find it hard to let go of their possessions, while some of the poorest people in the world can be incredibly generous and giving. I remember many times when I worked as a photographer and travelled through poorer areas of the world, such as pockets of Central Asia, Bhutan, India, China and Tibet, the people were incredibly generous to me. I would often be invited into homes for tea. In Uzbekistan, whenever I took someone's photo at a market, they would give me something back in exchange as a thank-you. I received plastic belts, knives, satchels of paprika, lemony cakes and even a free meal! These little gifts and generous acts of warmth made me feel safe as well as happy travelling in an unfamiliar country where very few people spoke English.

On the flip side I once hired an upscale yoga centre in Mexico to teach a retreat. While there they started charging us for additional small things they did not include in the general cost: internet was an extra twenty US dollars per person per week. A spare key for a room was five dollars more. My husband, who is an acupuncturist, asked if one of the therapists at the centre might have a few needles he could use. Later that day, five needles appeared in an envelope under our door with an invoice for twenty dollars; in London five needles normally cost him fifty pence. Every time they added a bill, my heart tightened. I felt sad that they did not feel enough abundance in their lives to help or offer services that were already there. In the end their lack of generosity made me lose my appreciation for the place. After leaving, despite it being a beautiful centre located on an idyllic beachfront, I never wanted to go back.

XIU YANG FOR CULTIVATING A GENEROUS LIFE

My father used to tell us that we will have many occasions throughout the day where we can choose between being petty and being generous in our actions. His sound advice was to always choose being generous. When we did this, we would then naturally learn to avoid pettiness. Try applying this choice throughout your day. This can be with gifts, money, attention, time or forgiveness. When you notice yourself at a crossroads – for example, someone has made a mistake and you're frustrated, angry and hugely inconvenienced. They apologise, but you want to make it known how upset you are. A potentially petty response would be to make them feel even worse about their errors, and to list all the ways they have inconvenienced you. A generous response would be to say, 'I accept your apology, but please understand this has made it hard for me today.'

CI BEI (慈悲): COMPASSION

The Chinese, Buddhist and yogic ideas of compassion are beautiful concepts to cultivate in how you choose to be in the world. To be compassionate is, in the words of my meditation teacher Martin Aylward, 'to stand in solidarity' with the suffering of another being. It is about seeing a difficult situation and feeling our heart come alive with a response that is clear, gentle and caring.

The reality is that being compassionate may not always be intuitive or easily forthcoming. Say, for example, you show up to work and find that your co-worker is grumpy. You might easily judge that person and become frustrated rather than compassionate towards them for having an 'off' day. Compassion can also be easily misconstrued as commiseration or a sign that you are somehow weak and too easily affected by other people's feelings. When you hear a sad or difficult story, for example, you can sometimes feel like you are being sucked into a depressed state. You may also feel compelled to start sharing your own hard-luck situation, or be inclined to offer unsolicited advice to try to help them fix their dilemma. None of these responses is truly compassionate.

Compassion is not about feeling pulled down by the suffering of others, but is about recognising someone else's difficulty as something you, too, have experienced or can understand. Knowing suffering as a universal truth becomes a source of compassion and deep insight. You can begin to see that no one gets to the end of their life without pain and loss. When you see that your pain is not just an individual burden, but a human quality we all share, you can begin to find ways to see dignity in yourself and in others. Learning to acknowledge your pain and the pain of others takes time and patience. Learning to open up to this pain takes even more courage and resources. This is why compassion must be a practice that you gradually and gently cultivate.

慈悲

The Chinese word for compassion is the compound *ci bei* (慈悲). The joining of these two words elicits layers of meaning to help us understand the nuance and depth of this concept. The first word, *ci* (慈), means kindness. It is comprised of the symbol for the heart (*xin* 心) beneath the character for 'here' (*zi* 兹). This implies that being kind is to be present with the heart. The second word, *bei* (悲), means sadness. *Bei* has the radical '非' (*fei*) on top, which means wrong, and on the bottom is also heart (*xin* 心). Compassion is therefore being fully present with kindness when the heart has been wronged.

As we explored in Chapter 10, the heart in Chinese is the *xin*, which is more than just the centre for our emotions: it also has a psychological role. Unlike the mind alone, the *xin* has the capacity to hold a wide range of complex and uncertain experiences. It is therefore the perfect place to meet suffering compassionately.

XIU YANG FOR LIVING A
COMPASSIONATE LIFE

The Buddha taught that to develop compassion, or *karuna*, we can explore our capacity for extending compassion at the personal, political and social levels of the human condition. Acts of compassion do not have to be grandiose. They can be simple and small, such as saying hello to a troubled neighbour or being available to talk if a friend needs a sounding board for a tricky situation. There is a helpful meditation on cultivating compassion that is similar to the *mettā* meditation on care shared in Chapter 10. Instead of the wish for happiness, health, safety and peace, you wish for freedom from pain and suffering for yourself and others. It is a similar idea to *mettā* but phrased in a way that acknowledges and opens you up to the existence of difficulty in the world.

THE PRACTICE: Start with visualising someone you know who is having a hard time. This could be someone who has just lost a loved one, been diagnosed with illness, has a hard time at work, or is going through a difficult break-up. Make sure this is a real person and someone you can relate to. Then begin to send them compassion, mentally saying the phrase, 'May you be free of your sorrow, sadness and pain.' Repeat this to yourself for a few minutes. From there, move on to extending this wish to yourself, then to a person you do not particularly like or find challenging/difficult, and then to all beings. Spend a few minutes on each person, moving at a pace that feels natural. It may take you longer to feel genuine compassion for some people than others so, in these cases, keep it simple and gentle. Also meet any resistance towards yourself for your own difficulties with compassion. If you feel your heart feels heavy, or starts to quiver or ache, know that this is a normal and natural part of the practice. Stay with the feeling and soften into your breath. Remind yourself that all human beings share pain. Touch into this shared experience – the connections, oneness and totality that underlie all life. When we open to this and sense interconnection and wholeness, we can discover a deep and lasting source of happiness and joy.

A Tibetan Girl's Disabled Hands:
A Story of Compassion

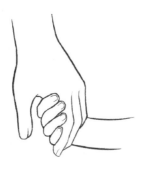

Dolma Wangmo was eleven years old in the spring of 2018 when she travelled from the remote mountains of China's Western Qinghai Province to see the ocean for the first time. Dolma Wangmo arrived in Yantai, on China's north-eastern seafront, with her adoptive grandfather and eight other Tibetan children and their parents. They all came as part of a medical mission my husband and I sponsor called the Glow Fund. The Glow Fund helps children with severe disabilities receive operations from leading orthopaedic surgeons from Stanford University's Lucile Packard Children's Hospital. The surgeons arrive in Yantai ready to evaluate the kids and operate on them within a week. Dolma Wangmo had a disability in her hands. When she was two years old, she suffered a viral infection that led to her whole body being paralysed for a year. She eventually regained motor control to most of her body, but her hands were left badly damaged. One hand was completely limp, and the other hand was contorted and difficult to use. Often people in China with disabilities have a much harder time finding regular work. Receiving an operation would not only potentially give her a fuller use of her hands, but would also give her better career opportunities in life.

On the day Dolma Wangmo had her consultation, there was chaos in the hospital: hundreds of other children had been invited that day to be seen by the specialists. Amidst the crowd, I saw her talking with one of the doctors. When they finished speaking, she stood up and walked away. I could tell by her slumped shoulders and downcast gaze that the news wasn't great. I asked her what the doctor said. When she lifted her gaze to see me, she immediately burst into tears and began to wail uncontrollably. She wasn't receiving the operation.

Her sobbing was attracting the attention of everyone in the waiting area, and my husband recommended I take her back into her hospital room. I wrapped my arms protectively around her and pushed our way through the crowd. We found her adoptive grandfather waiting for us. He had tears in his eyes. Seeing him, her crying grew louder and more piercing.

Then she broke my heart: she began to hit her hands. She hated them. When hitting them did no good, she started to try to shake them violently off of her arms. A Chinese nurse had come in to help. Her face was anguished, and she was crying. In response to Dolma Wangmo, she did what many might think to do when seeing someone suffering. She told her to stop crying. 'Bu yao ku! Bu yao ku!' she demanded. 'Stop crying! Stop crying!' Dolma Wangmo just cried louder. My response was to wrap my arms around her even tighter. I wanted to protect her. I told her I understand, that it's OK to cry, and if I were her I would be devastated and crying too.

In the days leading up to the consultation, I had seen what a clever, bubbly and mischievous girl she was despite having quite a tough life. She was an orphan who lost both of her parents in a car crash when she was three. The man she calls her grandfather took her in and cared for her. I imagined how many fantasies she must have spun in her mind about what an operation might do to get rid of her deformities and give her a chance at a normal life. Given her situation, her shame, self-loathing and self-inflicted violence were even more heartbreaking.

The spell of despair broke when her adoptive grandfather, who was standing on the other side of me, reached across to her. He took her small hands between both of his, and immediately began to kiss them. Tears mixed with his tender and poignant love. In that moment he became a saint; seeing her suffering, he extended her the immeasurable gift of compassion.

Fortunately, we were able to find a way to give Dolma Wangmo a successful operation for one of her hands. Through regular physical therapy she has also regained greater motor control in both of her hands. Her story nevertheless serves as a reminder of the importance of compassion towards others but also towards ourselves. We have all been in a situation like Dolma Wangmo; we have felt ashamed of our bodies or actions, hated ourselves, wished that we were different. But what if instead of turning that shame on ourselves or lashing out at others, we were able to respond with compassion towards the difficulty we face? I like to remind my students of this when I teach yoga classes. Occasionally, I have shared this story, and I ask students to think of their version of a grandfather who can kiss their hands when they feel frustrated by their bodies, ability or practice. When we learn to see the ways we experience difficulty and extend compassion towards our own experience, we can begin to see how suffering plays out in others, and perhaps learn to extend the gift of compassion to the world.

THE MAINTENANCE OF VIRTUES

Remember that xiu yang is a steady process. As such, it's unlikely that you will one day wake up feeling humane, generous and compassionate and never look back again. Just as a garden needs regular thinning, pruning and fertilising of the soil, keep regularly tending to the ways that keep your virtues healthy and growing day after day, and year after year. In this way you can continually refine and strengthen your foundations for happiness in the world.

13

Fluidity and Humility

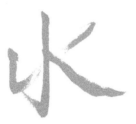

The patterns of our lives mirror the patterns of the universe, which are never fixed and always moving. These patterns ebb and flow like the Dao, which is most closely associated with the element of Water: humble with its ability to nourish all life without ever requiring anything in return. Water was also believed to be present at the beginning and end of all things, which again is like the Dao. We touched on this relationship in Chapter 1; here, we will expand on and explore the ways in which our relationship to nature and the Dao can also be a rich resource for living in the world.

MOVING WITH THE RIVER

How can we invite fluidity into our way of living through xiu yang? To start we must remember that xiu yang is never achieved by wilfulness or forcing a situation to be different from what it is. Say, for example, you have been growing roses in your garden for years, but, as they grow, a pine tree's increasing height starts to shade the roses from the sun. Trying to continue to grow roses in the shade would be like trying to force an impossible situation, as without sun the roses will struggle and wither. Better to choose a new flower to grow there, such as geraniums, which can thrive in the shade, and pick a nice new sunny spot where planting roses will ensure their beauty can flourish.

With xiu yang and fluidity you start from where you are and work with what you have. The Chinese have a phrase for this, which is *sui he* (隨河). *Sui he* means to move with the river. It means that rather than swim upstream and risk becoming grumpy and easily frustrated, you flow with the currents of life's ongoing change.

Being fluid can be natural in some situations, such as when you're excited to eat sushi with your friend but then she calls up and says she'd really rather eat pizza. To be *sui he* in other situations can be trickier. When we are sick, we usually try to resist being sick. Instead of fighting your body's need for recuperation by continuing to do all the things you normally do when you are healthy, use xiu yang's emphasis on cultivating the qualities of being *sui he:* flow into being sick! This means taking the time to care for yourself and nurture your body back to health. This may mean you take a day off work, but it saves you having to plod through five days of headaches, coughs and sniffles while on the job. If you are heartbroken, you gently turn towards your pain rather than forcing yourself into thinking you should bounce back straight away and be happy. This might initially feel more difficult, but in the long run it is better than turning away from pain and potentially allowing it to fester or trigger deeper levels of physical or emotional trauma and sadness. When you make room for your emotions to be seen, this allows them to move on and pass through you more thoroughly and quickly. Cultivating fluidity therefore starts with a willingness to meet whatever is here and go with the flow – however easy or difficult that might be.

BEING WITH OUR FLUID NATURE

The early Daoists believed that the body – including our blood, bones, energy, thoughts and spirit – is all part of the fluid, watery matrix that is the Dao.[90] We are a system of rivers, tributaries, pools and streams that move, ebb and flow. We are never the same person from one second to the next.

The currents that flow through our body help us to stay supple, but they also maintain our basic, fundamental functioning as an organism. Approximately 70 per cent of the body is fluid. This fluid flows through your joints, for example, helping with shock absorption as synovial fluid, and surrounds your organs as periorgan fluid. It exists as your blood, lymph and liquid between your cells (interstitial fluid). We even have fluid in our bones; rather than being dry and brittle, 50 per cent is actually made of a shock-absorbing gel formed by a mix of water and a chemical known as citrate. Despite these amazing fluids sustaining and maintaining our body's structure and function, much of the time we may feel anything but supple and fluid. This can be true in our bodies, but also true in the way we meet life experiences mentally and emotionally. Very often, when things go wrong, we stiffen, tighten and feel resistance to what is happening.

What can you do to support a fluid way of meeting the challenges of life when you feel stuck, stagnant or resistant? For starters you can draw on your fluid, watery body. Very often we move the body in sharp, sudden or jerky ways. Think of jumping jacks or military-style push-ups. When you shift to seeing your body as home to mostly fluids, your whole being has the potential to soften, including any tense or edgy mental and emotional state. Softening into your body's watery matrix can be a first step towards dissolving the hard, jagged tendencies of the mind.

Also, remember that the water in your body is one of the strongest yet softest elements in nature. The *Dao De Jing* describes how, 'Nothing in the world is as soft and yielding as water, yet for dissolving the hard and inflexible, nothing can surpass it.'[91] Water carves canyons through which rivers flow and can polish the most jagged rock into smooth stone. When you tune in to this quality, you can sense into the strength inherent in water that patiently wears down a stone's sharp edges and recognise that it can do the same to resistance in our bodies, minds, hearts or lives. This strength coupled with softness can become something we cultivate to meet whatever unfolds in our world with a gentle yet enduring dignity.

EXERCISE OF XIU YANG FOR FLUIDITY IN DAILY LIFE

The next time you begin to feel resistance from a friend, partner or colleague, tap into your watery self. Notice the way resistance feels in you physically. Do you feel it as tightness in your jaw? Chest? Or belly? Imagine the rivers of your body flowing, which can sustain and carry the rivers of your emotions and mental states. What are the ways in which you can let the soft strength of water help you meet this resistance and feel more fluid and free?

MOVING FLUIDLY

'Fluid' yoga practices, such as vinyasa flow, also support the natural movements of the body. The emphasis on the steady presence of breath in vinyasa allows you to begin to connect to a cycle that is similar to other natural, ongoing rhythms, such as the changing phases of the moon, the rising and setting of the sun, tidal movements or the turning of the seasons. These natural rhythms are easily lost to people living in cities, but this could explain why vinyasa flow is so popular and impactful today. It grants space to reconnect to an inner rhythm that is also reflected in the outer world.

From a Daoist viewpoint harmonising the fluids and energies of our minds and bodies allows us to become one with the flowing energies of nature and the universe. Over time and through experimentation, Daoists found the most effective way to do this was through fluid, gentle movements and smooth, deep breathing. These practices became what is known today as qigong. With qigong there is an emphasis on moving through the physical forms in a way that lets us feel carried by invisible currents of water. Our arms and hands are often described as being capable of dancing at the ends of rainbows, pushing waves or separating clouds. With qigong there is also an intention to soften rather than tense against the areas of the body that are tight and contracted. All of this helps bring a quality of fluidity into our daily life. In psychology this is known as the 'flow state'.[92] When we become completely absorbed in the task at hand, our hard work results in feeling focused, immersed and in the zone rather than frustrated and depleted. In this state the sense of ego dissolves and we find a way to move with experience that is happier, more fluid and free. This state is similar to the concept in Daoism known as *wu wei*, or effortless effort, described in Chapter 1.

THE DRAMA THAT INTERRUPTS FLUIDITY

Often our capacity for naturalness and fluidity is camouflaged by worry, tension and fear. This makes us feel far away from our natural way of being. Human beings seem inclined to make a bigger deal out of a naturally unfolding process than is required. Weather will change from sunny skies to rain, but, especially in the UK, our response to these normal fluctuations is to be excited by sun and saddened by rain. Similarly, success and failure are both natural processes, but we can easily overrate our success and beat ourselves up when we fail. A fluid meeting of these experiences would be to enjoy the sunshine when it's sunny without hoping it lasts forever, and appreciate the rain when it rains rather than wishing it were sunny. Similarly we can appreciate our successes in life when they arise without making them into standards we must always achieve, while also valuing our failures as opportunities to learn rather than turning them into deep doubts about our own capacity or self-worth. When we learn to meet all experience more fluidly, we can learn to live in harmony with the natural unfolding of experience without the tyranny of additional drama.

CULTIVATING HUMBLE QUALITIES

The heart of classical Chinese thinking extols the merits and strengths of being humble. In part, this reflects another quality of water when in balance: it always flows to the lowest places and, when available, follows the gentlest path. The root of the word humility is derived from the Latin word *humilis*, meaning 'low'. Because xiu yang aims to harmonise and align us with the Dao, this has meant that in ancient China leaders, scholars, officials and sages sought to emulate the qualities of water and the Dao by being subtle, modest and unassuming. In fact, those who pursued greatness, fame and fortune were never esteemed. Rather, a true sage, the *Dao De Jing* tells us, 'avoids excess, extravagance and arrogance' and 'does not brag, and so has merit … does not boast, and so endures …'[93]

In the West being humble is also generally considered to be a positive character trait. Saint Augustine defined humility as the root of all virtues, and Christ is often described in the Bible as meek and gentle of heart. But in today's competitive and individualistic society, cultivating humility is not always so straightforward. We live in a world that places a strong emphasis on personal achievement, class, success and standing out from the crowd. There is often an expectation to prove ourselves and show our accomplishments. To get a job we must demonstrate what we have achieved in our past. To market ourselves successfully we feel pressure to be sophisticated, clever, outgoing or funny. In the yoga world many teachers feel a need to show their physical abilities on social media platforms in order to attract students and followers. Left unchecked these tendencies to validate who we are can grow into thorny brambles of hubris or narcissism.

The opposite is also true: we can have such a strong aversion to boasting that we downplay ourselves and are left feeling deflated. We can end up resentful of those who naturally highlight their achievements or become frustrated that people do not see what we have done.

Both tendencies do not help free your heart and mind or let you live more happily in the world. When understood and cultivated in the right ways, humility is a reminder of the importance of living naturally and simply, like the sun that can rise perfectly above the earth and spread light in an easy and relaxed way across the land. It stresses that as much as we may think otherwise, our achievements are not the result of being an outstanding or amazing individual. Rather, it is often down to fortune, chance, upbringing, access, circumstances, privilege or kindness from others who have helped us along the way that we have achieved what we have in life. If we are good at something, it is often the by-product of many circumstances beyond our control. I often think about the fact that my parents were fortunate to leave China in 1949 and move to Taiwan, where they then had the opportunity to study overseas and emigrate to the United States. My cousins, who were left in China and subject to decades of Communist rule and the chaos of the Cultural Revolution, were not so fortunate. As a result, their lives in China were much harder than ours growing up in America. When we recognise that we rarely accomplish anything on our own, we can be humbled by the truth of our circumstances.

Humility also asks us to serve and support others where we can out of our love and care rather than out of a need or want. Seeing others happy is enough reward for our actions. We do our work not because we want to achieve greatness, but because we want to make a positive difference in our family, workplace or community. Seeing the beneficial results of our work should be enough to nourish us without the need for outside accolades and praise. We do what we can to reach out and inform people about who we are or what we do because we believe that what we share will in some way uplift, encourage or inspire them to change their perspective, mood or even course of life. We offer this freely without need for anything in return. This is how we can cultivate authentic humility in our lives.

When we focus our work on bettering the world in some way – whether that be through a smile, sharing a funny post on Facebook, volunteering for a charity or risking our lives to report on political upheaval – we do this while curbing our need for affirmation, attention and praise. This path of humility can help us create a much happier relationship with the world and how we live in it. In yoga this path is known as the balance of steady practice and letting go.[94] It is not that we don't make efforts to do well in life and strive towards positive achievements. Rather, we do what we need to, and then release our desire for a certain outcome. Or, in the words of the *Dao De Jing*, you 'do your work, then step back. The only path to serenity.'[95]

WHAT WE CAN LEARN FROM HUMILITY

There is much wisdom that can be learned from cultivating humility in our actions. From the perspective of practising xiu yang for a happier place in the world, these four ideas can help orientate us in living a more humble life.

- **HUMILITY DEEPENS OUR REVERENCE AND RESPECT FOR NATURE.** Rather than believing that human beings have a special place in the world or even the right to dominate it, humility reminds us that we are part of nature, and nature is part of us. This enables us to develop a respect for and deeper appreciation of nature and its mystery, beauty and power. It also allows us to embrace the idea of impermanence and ongoing change: all things arise, dissolve and re-emerge in perfectly natural ways.

- **HUMILITY HELPS US DO WORK THAT IS IN THE SERVICE OF OTHERS.** All great saints tell us to serve others. There is a common message in spiritual practices: don't think about yourself, think of others. Yet you must always remember that to serve others you must first feel your own heart full and capable of giving out generously and freely. This is why xiu yang for your body, mind, heart and world are equally important. When you work on all aspects of yourself, you feed the vehicle of life (your body), the root of life (your energy), the spirit of life (your heart and mind) and the domain of life (the world) until all aspects are energised, healthy and able to bring about positive change.

- **HUMILITY CURBS YOUR NEED AND WANT FOR MORE.** Once I interviewed a Bhutanese nun, who told me, 'Contentment is the supreme of all wealth.' In today's commercially driven world, we can easily become trapped into seeking happiness through material gain or a desire for more recognition and praise. Humility helps you realise that you have enough and that you are enough. So long as you are fed, sheltered, healthy and in a good community, you can be happy. While sometimes buying new things can feel good, just as a promotion can make us feel proud, recognise that these little comforts are momentary types of happiness. Humility guides you towards seeing the possibility for a lasting joy and ease that are free from the traps of wanting and demanding more.

- **HUMILITY HELPS YOU SOFTEN YOUR NEED TO BE RIGHT.** When you give up the need to be right, you humble yourself to the views and opinions of others. By letting down the guard of self-righteousness, your defences soften and you can begin to listen to others more fully. While you may not agree with what they are saying, at least you can open your heart and mind to another person's way of seeing things. Through an openness to ideas you cultivate a more generous way of being that makes room for new ideas. This keeps you curious, open and free.

OUR PLACE IN THE NATURAL WORLD

There is an inherent belief in classical Chinese thinking that human beings play a relatively unimportant and small role in our relationship to the vast, mysterious powers and nature of the universe. To be humble is to remember this relationship and position in the universe. It's an idea that is often depicted in Chinese scroll paintings. One of the Song Dynasty's most famous painters, Fan Kuan, represented the idea that nature is large and dominant in comparison to the human being. In one of his best-known works, *Travellers Among Mountains and Streams*, people are depicted as tiny figures that can easily be missed amidst the towering mountains, thick trees and flowing river surrounding them.

The classical Chinese view of humility sees humans as holding no special place on earth. We are simply one manifestation of the qi, or energy, that is part of all existence. In a sense this perspective opens us up to a freedom to live our lives with a respect for nature and a trust in the cycles of creation and dissolution. We simply arise from the Dao and return to it, which is what all living things in the world experience.

CULTIVATING HUMILITY

Humility was seen as a process, practice and outcome of meditation as well as a means of experiencing oneness with the Dao. By working with the meditation and mindfulness practices in Part 1 and 2 of this book, humility will naturally arise. To cultivate humility through practice and embrace it as a process, you can work with these three additional exercises and ideas.

1. **SOAK THE SUCCESS INTO YOUR OWN BONES.** The next time you achieve something or seek recognition for a job well done, let the success soak into your own being. See what it is like not to share your accomplishment or recognition with someone else. See what it is like not to hope for praise, but instead feel gladdened by the results themselves if they affect others, or simply feel this accomplishment nourish your own heart.

2. **REPEAT LINES FROM CLASSICAL DAOIST TEXTS.** I carry a pocket-sized copy of the *Dao De Jing* with me in my bag. Often I will read a few lines from it as a reminder of the importance of humility as well as how to find contentment in simple ways. Some of my favourite verses on humility that I often read and repeat are these:[96]

   - Chapter 8: 'The supreme good is like water, which nourishes all things without trying to. It is content with the low places that people disdain. Thus it is like the Dao.'

   - Chapter 22: 'Because he does not display himself, people can see his light. Because he has nothing to prove, people can trust his words.'

   - Chapter 66: 'All streams flow to the sea because it is lower than they are. Humility gives it its power.'

3. **MAKE YOURSELF A LIGHT.**[97] In a poem by Mary Oliver titled 'The Buddha's Last Instruction', she describes how, before he died, the Buddha chose to speak these words. The Buddha could have said anything, but in choosing this he quietly asks us to do what we can in the world to make it a better place.

Humility can be like this: at times it can make us feel small and inconsequential in the world. Yet within each of us is the ability to effect positive change in our own ways. To me there is a beautiful quality to humility: the ability to do great things without needing to be more than a light for ourselves and others.

As a way to cultivate the most positive qualities of humility, remind yourself throughout your day of the ways – large or small – that you can make of yourself a light.

14

Spontaneity and Creativity

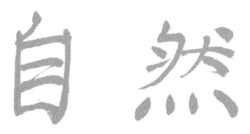

Daoist sages since antiquity embraced the notion of spontaneity. To them spontaneity was a quality that arose when we felt creative, natural and free. The word for spontaneity in Chinese is *zi ran* (自然), which translates as nature, or the world of animals, plants and the universe, but it also means 'true to oneself'. In Daoism to be true to oneself is to remember that we are part of nature and its unfolding. This view assumes that spontaneity and creativity are natural energies that arise like the Dao: uncontrived, instinctive and free.

This ancient viewpoint is one embraced by many clinical psychologists today, such as Dr Max Hammer and Dr Barry Hammer, the former a distinguished psychology professor who helped found the Clinical Psychology department at the University of Maine. In a 2015 article published in the *Journal of Psychology and Clinical Psychiatry* called 'The Enhancement of Spontaneity and Creativity', Hammer describes how creativity and spontaneity are the results of simplicity and 'natural integrity'; they can never be pursued or contrived.[98] He argues that spontaneity and creativity therefore arise in us when the controlling process of the ego subsides and we no longer see ourselves as separate from the wider world around us.

When we feel part of a totality and wholeness that is always present, the momentum behind our ego slows down. This idea lies at the heart of xiu yang and the Dao. When you learn to feel more free and easy in the world, your capacity to live creatively and spontaneously awakens.

THE SPONTANEOUS LIFE: FREEDOM FROM EXTREMES

Zhuangzi, one of Daoism's most renowned ancient sages, was one of spontaneity's greatest champions. Accessing a spontaneous life did not mean becoming impulsive and reckless in behaviour, for this would mean giving in to our obsessions, habits and whims. Rather, Zhuangzi advocated living simply and free from the extremes of right and wrong, good and bad, and other burdens of opinion that create separation, boundaries and disagreements among people.[99] When we let go of our need to be right, the ego's demands soften their grip, letting our hearts feel more carefree and easy.

Living with simplicity and refraining from having terse arguments about right or wrong opinions may sound good, but having structures, ideas, knowledge and opinions has also served us well. In many ways these qualities define us as human beings. Contention and debate enable us to have dialogue, leading to innovation and growth. We are rational thinking creatures. Is living spontaneously and free from views and opinions possible or even desirable?

To forget ideas we must first learn them. To let go of opinions we must first acquire them. To cultivate an attitude of spontaneity and freedom we can apply the art of xiu yang by taking the time to know things deeply. This means educating yourself, but also seeing things from both sides, expanding your view beyond your own opinions, and reaching across the aisle to create common ground. To do this we can look to the Buddha's teachings on 'right speech', which is the cultivation of language that unites, creates goodwill and mutual benefit rather than division or blame.[100] We can also remember Zhuangzi's warning that 'words and actions are like wind and waves. They can stir up a storm at a moment's notice' and 'lead to rash decisions'.[101] Best to be concerned with the things that nourish you, Zhuangzi reminds us, and stay away from things that cause harm.

In the 2016 US presidential elections I remember very clearly the day the results were announced and Donald Trump was elected president. My husband and I were in China for the charity we run, the Glow Fund. We were with Stanford University surgeons who were performing orthopaedic operations for Chinese orphans and children from Tibetan regions. The wife of one of the surgeons voted for Trump, whom we did not expect to win the election. All of us that day were shocked, sad and confused, but we refrained from expressing our opinions while in his company. In fact, one doctor, who is Jewish and was a child during the Second World War, gave context: we do not know what will happen, he cautioned, so we can only carry on and do the best work we can today. Though we wanted to express our feelings, each of us also knew that angry words would only make an important member of our team, who loved his wife and supported her views, feel separate and judged. Looking back on that day, the doctors all showed good xiu yang: they chose unity despite the heated sentiment of division and separation. In their own way they made a difference in one person's life, and became examples of how the wisdom of *Inward Training* could be revealed today:

> *Those who can transform even a single being—*
> *We call them 'spiritual'.*
> *Those who can alter even a single situation,*
> *We call them 'wise'.*

Inward Training (Neiye), Chapter 9[102]

To begin living with the spontaneity and freedom of the Dao we are invited to use techniques to help us step away from assumptions, judgements and other actions that create friction, discord and division. In this way we can live more naturally and spontaneously in the world. We also invoke the inherent goodness of the Dao, whose infinite and effulgent source feeds everything between heaven, earth and beyond.

XIU YANG FOR FREE AND SPONTANEOUS LIVING: LISTENING TO FIND COMMON GROUND

In the midst of discussion, argument, heated conversation or debate where you may feel unheard, frustrated or talked over, get curious. Look around. Go inside and feel. 'Un-mind' your mind. Dissolve the need to feel heard. Let your opinion soften. Then begin to listen deeply. This is the springboard of reflective, wise response.

What is the person trying to say? Can you understand their perspective? Especially if you see their opinion as extreme or aggressive, what can you say that unites rather than divides? This can be as ordinary and simple as talking about the weather, or something levelling upon which you both agree. Look for the common ground you share, not the differences. A sudden change of topic may also soften their defences and allow them the space to unclench from the grasp of their strong opinion. Then choose words that nourish: 'How can we create better understanding between us?' or, 'I'd like to make an effort to genuinely hear you.'

Most of the time this is hard. But if you can learn to temper your frustration by listening deeply, your tendencies to lash out can be curbed. This gives you the possibility to respond with greater wisdom, love and compassion. These qualities triumph over ignorance and slowly transform our tendencies towards misunderstandings, anger or pain into understanding.

Therefore, as best you can, in any situation, try to understand before being understood. Reach across the table and use words that calm the storm.

XIU YANG FOR UNITY

This is a practice based on one I first learned from Erich Schiffmann. It is premised on the fact that most of the time, when we walk down the street, we see a person and immediately categorise them as tall, short, old, young, good-looking or strange-looking. Rather than having these categories define a person in our mind, we can learn to become *faster* than our conditioning by intervening in making these judgements. Instead of labelling the people we see in this automatic way, we can practise saying to ourselves 'brother', 'sister' or 'friend' as we walk by a person. I do this practice regularly. Once, when I was on my way to teach a yoga class in central London, someone cut me off on the street. My first impulse was to curse at them and call them a nasty name. Instead, I labelled him 'brother'. Immediately I felt my anger soften. I also felt more connected to his insensitivity and rudeness, saw his rushing as a human trait. They are qualities I recognise only too well in myself.

The next time you are somewhere where there are a lot of people, at a busy airport, museum or café, try to get faster than your conditioning. Instead of labelling someone as handsome, which can be a compliment but also sets up the expectation that another person is less attractive, see that person instead as a brother, sister or friend. Label them as you walk by: 'brother', 'brother', 'friend', 'sister', 'sister', 'friend', and remember that we are all part of a whole.

STAYING IN
BEGINNER'S MIND

One way to help us free ourselves and touch into our natural spontaneity is to remain as much as we can in the Zen Buddhist mindset known as *shoshin*, or 'beginner's mind'. Shunryu Suzuki describes how 'in the beginner's mind there are many possibilities, but in the expert's there are few'.[103] When we are a beginner in a certain area, we can feel worried and insecure about our grasp of material. I often see this uncertainty in new students to my yoga and qigong classes. Many are concerned about looking right and doing the postures 'correctly'. What I tell them is to enjoy being a beginner and learning something new. I also often remind my whole class, which will frequently be a mix of beginners as well as more advanced practitioners and teachers, that cultivating beginner's mind is actually the most advanced practice!

When we think we know the best or right way, we limit ourselves by cutting off our possibilities and readiness to meet anything – whether it is easy or challenging. 'Knowing mind', or thinking we are an expert at something, becomes a very narrow place to be. Answers are dead ends. In beginner's mind there is the potential to experience things as new and different. As Erich Schiffmann likes to say, 'Look without knowing and see what you see.' Seeing things with fresh eyes helps us remain open to life's mysteries and infinite possibilities.

Developing this beginner's mind can be a bit tricky at first, as much of the time our patterns of behaviour are well established. In yoga and Buddhism these patterns are known as *samskaras*, or conditioned ways of being. Some *samskaras* are helpful, such as brushing your teeth twice a day. Other habits are not so useful, such as indulging in food, drugs, alcohol or shopping during stressful times. Practices in yoga and Buddhism are designed to bring the light of awareness to these patterns. When we begin to see our habit patterns, we have a chance to consider whether these behaviours are useful or destructive.

We can keep the useful patterns, and work to gradually undo and change the harmful ones.

Whether it is a physical addiction like eating cake twice a day, or a tendency to snap at our children or partners, cultivating a change in our responses takes time and steady attention. This is why xiu yang is not a ten-step process to change. When we gradually work to effect these changes in our lives, we can look back after a few years and see the positive work that has taken place and transformed us.

CREATIVITY: OUT OF NOTHING COMES SOMETHING

In Chapter 4 we looked at the cycles of the seasons. We saw how winter in the Chinese Five Elements is the time of year when the earth lies fallow. With less obvious external activity happening in nature, bulbs, plants and trees drink in resources to their root systems and prepare themselves underneath the earth for the creative expressions and growth of spring. Winter is also the season associated with the element of Water, which is most like the Dao in that it underlies and gives birth to all life. Winter and water can therefore be seen as a source of creativity and potential.

For you to access the possibilities of water you can work towards slowing down and doing less. This is often counter to expectations from jobs and daily life, where we are expected to be productive and contribute 100 per cent of our efforts 100 per cent of the time. Yet if you look to the natural world, nature always takes its time to rest each autumn and winter. If it does not, then it loses its ability to bloom in the spring. You are the same. You need time to rest and recuperate, not only in your daily life, but also in accessing your deeper creative resources and potential over time.

When we are too busy, it can be hard to think through problems or feel inspired by new ideas. If you think back to a time when you stepped off the proverbial hamster wheel and were truly able to step away from the responsibilities of life and lie fallow, what was the feeling like by the end of your break? Did your time off give you fresh perspective or inspiration? Energy for coming back to 'real life'? The wherewithal to meet new challenges? We can often underestimate the importance of granting ourselves the space to do nothing.

The importance of substantial downtime is finding its way into certain sectors of the business world. It is championed by people in creative industries, such as the architect Stefan Sagmeister. Every seven years, Sagmeister closes his New York design studio for twelve months to rejuvenate and refresh his staff's creative ideas.[104] He says this proper rest and time off is what leads to creative innovation. Even with the additional cost of continuing to rent his studio and support his employees, it proved financially successful as the ideas generated from his staff during their sabbatical led to highly lucrative new projects. In fact, everything they designed in the seven years following the first sabbatical had originated in the year off. It turns out that doing nothing most likely gives you time to tap into the source of your creativity. Like the famous theory of the Big Bang, it can open you up to the possibility that out of nothing comes something incredible.

FIVE WAYS TO CULTIVATE SPONTANEITY AND CREATIVITY

1. Do nothing and lie fallow. Take a real break. Do this in your day by sitting outside without your phone or other people around. Lie on your bed, sit in a park, or soak in a bath without distractions like a book or music. If you can, do very little for an entire day. It will be a day well spent! On days you do not have much time, however, even five or ten minutes can be a valuable investment.

2. Practise the 'brother, brother, sister, sister, friend, friend' model when you are in a room of people or walking down the street.

3. Resist following structures and quick categorisations. Challenge certain orthodoxies. See beyond dualistic thinking of right and wrong. Explore freely. Look beyond convention.

4. Cultivate mindfulness daily. Think of mindfulness as developing creative responses to life. In time mindfulness will help you shift your patterns, or *samskaras*, and be more free.

5. Tap into your own feelings of expression. Engage in activities that let you freely express yourself, whether that be through music, poetry, art, dance, cooking or theatre. Be the singer not the song.

15

Spaciousness

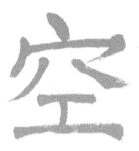

I remember being on a meditation retreat, where the teacher asked the group, 'What does your heart long for?' The first person who spoke said 'space'. This was also the answer in my mind. At the time I was feeling excited but also overwhelmed. I had finished teaching a retreat the previous weekend and had just begun packing up our house in London in preparation for a move to the countryside. On top of my normal classes and teacher training, I was also trying to rewrite a book proposal. Life's many demands had left my heart feeling overcrowded and overburdened, and craving space.

By design the heart naturally creates physical space whenever its chambers alternately empty and fill. Spaciousness is often what the heart longs for but lacks. When your heart feels spacious, you can be inspired, spirited and connected to your true self. You can embrace life and relax into knowing you have a rightful place in the world. But when the heart feels loaded and cramped, the light of the heart can begin to dim.

By practising xiu yang you start the invaluable work of cultivating the qualities of spaciousness that support your heart. This work ripples out and affects those in the field of your friends, family and communities in positive ways. You may also consider what the right space is for optimum growth and happiness in the world. This includes the space of your environment, but also the people and company with whom you choose to surround yourself.

CULTIVATING A SPACIOUS HEART AND MIND

Plants – like our heart – require space for their expansion and growth. If a pot is too small for a plant's roots, its development will be thwarted. Not only will it be hungry for more soil, but it becomes restricted, confined and unable to absorb the nutrients it needs to continue to grow. We can likewise feel uncomfortable in our own skin and suffocated if we do not have the required space to live and breathe freely.

In nature, however, plants do not grow in pots. They often have as much soil and space as is naturally allotted to them to flourish. Until recent levels of pollution threatened habitats, wild fish and birds similarly always enjoyed sufficient water and sky. The thirteenth-century Zen master Dogen wrote, 'When a fish swims, it swims on and on, and there is no end to the water. When a bird flies, it flies on and on, and there is no end to the sky. There was never a fish that ran out of water, or a bird that flew out of the sky.'[105] When thinking about this idea, I have found myself asking: what is it that humans have no end of? What makes us feel trapped, crowded and limited? And what can help us ensure we have the right space to live our lives fully?

What I believe we have an endless supply of is consciousness. Consciousness is vast and limitless. There is no end to our awareness, just as there is no confirmed limit to the sky and universe that expands around us in all directions. But so often we fixate not on the spaciousness of our experience, but on

194

the objects – which are our thoughts – that arise within them. This is similar to how we may walk into a room and see the objects in the room while entirely missing the space around the objects that allows them to be there. It is the way in which our hearts and minds meet experience that traps us into believing they are crowded and limited in nature.

Many spiritual traditions teach that the mind and heart are anything but tight and limited. How do we learn this? Through opening the doors of our perception and directing the mind and heart towards spaciousness whenever possible. One way to help this process is meditation. The philosopher J. Krishnamurti wrote that it is: 'In meditation, mind discovers space. Space is held within a room and there is space outside it. Is there a space which has no frontiers, which has no boundaries, and, therefore, no centre? This is meditation, to find out.'[106] Another idea illustrating that the mind and heart are far more open than we recognise comes from the 1950s writer Aldous Huxley. Huxley, who experimented with a number of psychedelic drugs in his time, also believed that the brain functions as a 'reducing valve', trickling in a tiny amount of our 'Mind at Large' to keep us alive.[107] Though drugs may play a part for some people to see this, for centuries the yogis, Buddhists and Daoist sages have mostly turned to other means, primarily lifestyle, breathing, meditation and the cultivation of the virtues we have explored in *Xiu Yang*.

Here are five practices that may help you cultivate qualities of spaciousness when your worldly burdens begin to crowd your heart and mind.

1. **OBSERVE THE SPACE AROUND AN OBJECT.** The next time you make a cup of coffee or tea, look at the cup. Then see the space around the cup. If the table were completely full, there would be no space available for the cup to be placed. Choose to see the space that makes the cup sitting on the table possible, and be thankful for it. As you drink your tea, notice how, as the liquid level lowers, more space

becomes available inside the cup. Observe the steam rising from the liquid, and how space allows the filling of the cup to be possible.

You can also do this type of exercise when you walk into a space or room full of people – maybe a restaurant, office or on a bus. Take note of everything that crowds the space in that room. Then pay attention to the space around those objects. The space is required for the objects to exist. We can always choose where to focus our attention: on the objects filling the room or the space around them.

2. **DURING THE DAY NOTICE WHEN YOUR MIND OR HEART FIXATES ON SOMEONE OR SOMETHING AND TIGHTENS.** Notice the thought, idea or person around which your mind or heart has tightened. Begin to see that a story or memory has arisen within the infinite spaciousness of your own consciousness. Choose to become aware of your consciousnesses that gave rise to the awareness, rather than the idea or thought itself.

3. **FOCUS ON YOUR HEART ALTERNATELY EMPTYING AND FILLING.** With each heartbeat visualise the chambers of your heart alternately moving between being spacious and full. Pay particular attention to the possibility for emptiness in your heart. Now focus on your breathing. Pause at the end of your exhale for a moment – it can be a second or longer than you think. In this pause feel the spaciousness before the in breath begins to fill the lungs again.

4. **STAND IN *WUJI* – EMPTINESS STANCE.** The qigong standing meditation form is called *Wuji*, or 'Emptiness Stance' (see Chapter 8, page 114) It also represents the primordial universe, which is boundless and infinite. Standing in *Wuji* is believed to establish a feeling of

undisturbed roots into the earth as well as an expansive connection to the primordial energy of the universe. In this state of emptiness you can cultivate inner steadiness and stillness like a mountain, yet also remain aware of the fluid changes happening at all times within your breath, mind, body and spirit. You can stand in *Wuji* for a few minutes or, with steady practice, as long as twenty, thirty or even sixty minutes.

5. **CLEAR, GATHER AND SEAL.** This is also a practice from qigong. You can do this after *Wuji*, or in any situation in your day. It involves using intention and slow, gradual movements in the arms and hands. Breathe naturally throughout the practice.

   • Begin with your hands at your sides, palms facing up. Imagine gathering what feels cramped, crowded and cluttered in your mind, heart or body. This can be physical tension or thoughts. Then start to raise the hands and arms slowly and gradually to the sides and overhead. When your arms and hands rise overhead, turn the palms towards the earth, middle fingers pointing towards each other. Bend the elbows, and slowly and gradually begin to lower the hands down in front of your face, throat, chest

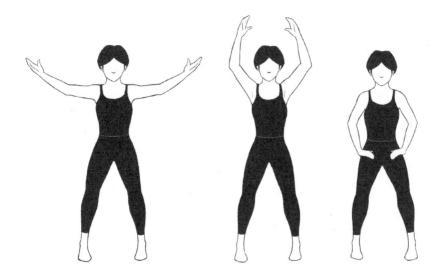

197

and belly. As you do this, use the hands to imagine clearing whatever you have just gathered that is cramping and crowding your experience out of the form of your body.

- Repeat this movement with a different intention to gather what feels spacious with your hands. Fill spaciousness into the areas you have cleared.

- Repeat for a third and final round, this time with the intention to gather the spaciousness you have filled into the form of your body, and seal it in. When you do this, seal it into a place in your body, mind and heart that can grow into insight and wisdom in how you meet the world.

MAKE SPACE FOR GOOD COMPANY

In nature potato and tomato plants thrive when in the company of their own species. Before pesticides and chemical fertilisers, traditional farming methods saw the value in planting a community of plants together to create beneficial partnerships and synergies. In permaculture, which emphasises a sustainable approach to agriculture using natural ecosystems, these partnerships are called 'guilds'. One classic guild from Native American farming is called the 'three sisters': corn, beans and squash.[108] They form a guild because each of these plants brings benefit and support to the others. The beans give nitrogen to the soil, which boosts the corn and squash. The corn becomes a trellis for the beans to climb, and the squash covers the ground with its broad leaves and keeps the soil cool and moist while also preventing weeds from coming up around the plants.

Plants can also benefit from a technique called 'companion planting' – clustering certain plants together to fend off pests and prey, as well as to achieve optimum growth. Coriander grows well with dill and anise, but will prevent fennel from forming seeds. When grown between rows of carrots and cabbage, coriander and dill protect carrots from predatory pests.[109] Companion planting has come back into use as more and more people embrace non-invasive and natural techniques of farming.

In the same way that plants seek good company, human beings have evolved to form families, tribes, villages, cities and societies for good reasons: strength in numbers means safety, as well as shared ideas, visions and goals. Like plants we thrive when nurtured and supported by the right people. The difficulty is that sometimes the people closest to us are our families, and we all know the complications of family life. As the Insight Meditation teacher Jack Kornfield often likes to say, 'That's why it's called a nuclear family.'[110]

As much as possible, choose to be around people who inspire you and let you feel most yourself. This is not always easy, but it is important. People who are bright, positive and radiate goodness have an infectious effect on others. I remember when my mother-in-law died unexpectedly. She was one of the most positive, thoughtful and infectiously cheerful people I knew. In fact, when my father heard the news, he said, 'She was someone who made everyone happy. Even just being in the same room with her always made me feel so good and so happy.'

When you surround yourself with good company, constructive transformation and change are far easier to accomplish. The Buddha knew this. This is why he placed as much emphasis on spiritual community – something he called *sangha* – as he did on spiritual teachings and the potential for each person to awaken. Though it can take time, it is never too late to find a community that helps you grow the best in yourself. As you build your family network (given or chosen), friendships and work relationships, consider how you might create 'guilds' in your life that offer each person a mutually beneficial relationship.

As you begin this type of xiu yang, ask yourself: who in your life encourages a good use of your resources? Who or what makes you feel that your energy and time are depleted? The right company can help you feel safe, but also give you space to blossom and mature into your truer, vibrant, happier you.

THE UPSIDE OF EMPTINESS

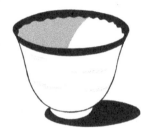

Often, when we think of something as being empty, we think of it as being deficient or lacking. A gas tank on empty is bad news. People who speak carelessly or break promises speak with 'empty words'. An empty seat at the table means someone we expected has not appeared. Yet in the Daoist and Buddhist concepts emptiness is the opposite. In Daoism emptiness is the space of potential. A cup needs to be empty so that you can fill it with a warm tea. As the *Dao De Jing* observes, 'We join spokes together in a wheel, but it is the centre hole that makes the wagon move; we hammer wood for a house, but it is the inner space that makes it liveable.'[111] In Buddhism emptiness, or *suññatā*, is the state where our scattered and confused mind sees past duality into the reality that, in the words of Zen teacher Thich Nhat Hanh, 'the one is in the all and the all is in the one.'[112] When you can see emptiness not as a negative concept but as what helps you see potential and the oneness of all experience, it will help you shift the way you approach any object, person or experience. Rather than narrowing your perception, this view of emptiness can help you feel qualities of immeasurable and boundless possibilities.

SPACIOUSNESS AND EQUANIMITY

With spaciousness there also arises the opportunity to cultivate the attitude and virtue of equanimity. Equanimity, or *upekkha* in both Sanskrit and Pali, is a central practice in Buddhist as well as yogic teachings. It is one of the four immeasurables, or *bhramavihara*.

Equanimity is a state where we feel even-minded and calm. Sometimes it can be conflated with notions of being indifferent, denying our feelings, or being distant and detached. Understood best, however, equanimity is a way of being that arises when you feel wide open and spacious. In this state you can begin to trust, meet and respond to life in a way that lets you care more deeply and fully about what truly matters. You make room within your heart for joy, pain, sorrow and challenges. You meet life in ways that neither oppose nor demand more from it. You remain steady, trusting and open to all of life.

When you cultivate equanimity, you develop the ability to stay calm, or even gracious, when difficulty arises. You begin caring deeply and feeling invested in a situation without becoming emotionally distraught or caught up in your habits and reactivity to situations. When you are in a calm and objective state, rather than in a distressed or overly involved position, you can best serve and help others. The last thing anyone would want is for an emergency medic to show up to the scene of an accident and panic.

Meditation is the perfect place to explore your capacity for equanimity. When you sit down to meditate, you will most likely experience dullness, sleepiness, impatience or discomfort. I can often track a wish to push some experience away or a desire for it to be different as I meditate. When you have the space to notice these things, there's an opportunity to notice and respond to them with the skill of kindness. When you pay attention to what offsets you in quiet sitting, you can explore the messy complexity of your experience, and be gentle or perhaps even humorous about it. You learn to allow for it and develop clarity around what your responses might be. You also begin to foster discernment, which allows you to differentiate between the thoughts and actions that help you and those that undermine your ease and peace.

With equanimity you begin to understand that all experience is simply experience. It is inherently neither good nor bad, but simply experience. You may like or dislike an experience, but this does not mean that the experience is inherently right or wrong. All of it is there. None of it is wrong to have. In this way you learn to soften the struggle against what you resist and what you wish would be different. You can see what you tend to push away, defend against, or demand to be a certain way, and sit with it.

This practice can readily translate into daily life. There have been occasions where I have watched my husband cut vegetables differently to how I would cut them. On the wrong day small differences like this can make me irritated, turn into a control freak and nag him. This only makes both of us suffer. By cultivating some spaciousness and an attitude of equanimity, I can take a moment to attend to what I am feeling. Before reacting on impulse, I might see that how he cuts vegetables is not that important and will not make that much of a difference to our long-term happiness. With equanimity I can allow for his approach. I can also ask myself: would I rather have him feel annoyed by me nagging him over vegetable cutting, or would I rather invest my energy and attention and time into loving him more, creating a sustainable relationship built on communication, mutual respect and understanding?

The spaciousness of equanimity allows you to begin to care for, respect and extend greater understanding to a situation rather than employing harshness and judgement. It can help you on personal levels but also be a call for how you might meet the many problems facing the wider world today. When you cultivate equanimity, you can be moved by injustice and become motivated to make things better without letting your deep inner serenity become disturbed.

With equanimity you also begin to open up and trust the magnificence, mystery and magic of life. You make room for the uncontrollable and unknowable to be as they are. Cultivating equanimity becomes a practice of radically accepting the world in a way that cares deeply and wishes to respond in the best possible way. This acceptance points you towards the possibility of meeting all of life, including its most vexing problems and polarising inconsistencies, with a generous, compassionate and open heart.

CONCLUSION

From Inner Balance to Outer Radiance

The simple beauty of xiu yang is that each act of self-cultivation helps us grow our resources for better health and long-term happiness. The instant you immerse yourself in these practices, you take one step closer towards inner balance. When you touch into this state, an outer radiance naturally shines through you. The authors of *Inward Training* spoke to this possibility when they wrote that with 'spirit, no one knows its limits; its luminosity extends to know the ten thousand beings'.[113]

While not every seed you plant will necessarily grow and flourish, what matters is your intention behind wishing to cultivate what is best in your life, which is also best for the world. By cultivating your body, mind, heart and world you emanate goodness into every corner of your mandala's squares and every sphere of your mandala's circles. While never easy, remembering that you are part of the natural, changing world invites you to feel sensitively into the rhythms of life and your responses to the world's complexities. This will help you step into a state of mind that is modest, curious and awake. It will also help you experience the vastness of being one human, living in a wide-open and ever-expanding universe.

In fifteen years of exploring xiu yang practices my outlook on health, love, life and the world has been reshaped and transformed in ways that have given me far greater hope for long-term happiness and balance. Mainly, they have helped me weather the joys and sorrows of life with far more grounding in myself and my relationships than I ever imagined possible. Throughout this process I have learned three things that I would like to offer in conclusion to this journey of xiu yang:

1. **TAKE TIME TO NURTURE AND CULTIVATE YOUR HEART.** Xiu yang requires gentle perseverance. Move slowly and resist impulses to rush through life. Much of xiu yang's work is reminiscent of seeds planted in the soil; it takes time and preparation for good crops to grow. Bide your time and maintain a willingness to cultivate the best in yourself patiently. This can be hard, especially when everything in the world seems to be increasing in speed, but remember that the heart thrives when steady and calm.

2. **CELEBRATE NATURE'S MYSTERY, VASTNESS AND RADIANCE.** When you look out from the top of a mountain or cast your gaze upwards to the stars at night, you can immediately sense into the mystery and vastness of what nature creates. Nature has and will continue to evolve and endure the test of time. It is inwardly balanced and outwardly radiant. As part of nature, you can look within yourself to find this same path to radiance.

3. **THE PULSATION OF THE DAO IS LOVE.** In a chaotic and imperfect world remember that all humans are fundamentally connected by the energy of love. When you meet life from your heart, even if it aches or feels shattered by loss, you will know this. Also, remember that each person, whether they know it or not, is striving towards a life where they can fear less and love more.

On a final note, remember that the landscape of your body, heart, mind and world is capable of producing incredible beauty. As you cultivate, let what you grow become vibrant and flourish. This will let you live wholeheartedly and in a way that positively impacts yourself, your community and the world. Each step you take will awaken the expansiveness of your heart. Light can shine out of anyone and anything. This is the gift of xiu yang: letting the mysterious and luminous quality of your heart be cultivated and nourished so that it can shine brighter.

ENDNOTES

Introduction: A Self that is Whole and Complete

1 Farhi, D., *Yoga Mind, Body and Spirit*, 2011. New York: Henry Holt and Company, p. 5.

2 Johnson, I., 'Are China's Rulers Getting Religion?', *New York Review of Books*, 29 October 2011. Available at https://www. nybooks.com/daily/2011/10/29/china-getting-religion/ [Accessed 3 August 2018].

3 See Bodhi, B., 'The Buddha and His Dhamma', 2006. Access to Insight. Available at https://www.accesstoinsight.org/lib/authors/ bodhi/wheel433.html [Accessed 25 October 2018].

Part 1: The Art of Xiu Yang

4 Quote by the artist Paul Chan, used to describe his goal in creating art, in Calvin Thompkins's article, 'The Shadow Player: The Provocations of Paul Chan', *The New Yorker*, 26 May 2008. Available at https://www.newyorker.com/magazine/2008/05/26/ shadow-player/ [Accessed 6 August 2018].

5 *Lao Tzu Tao Te Ching*, II.7, 1963. Translated by Mimi Kuo-Deemer.

6 *Inward Training (Neiye)*, Chapter 4. Translated by Louis Komjathy, 2008 (2003), in *Handbooks for Daoist Practice*, Vol. 1. Hong Kong: Yuen Yuen Institute, p. 32.

7 Lau, op cit, II.5, p. 58.

8 *The Yoga Sutrā of Patanjali*, II.33. Translation and commentary by Sri Swami Satchidananda, 2010 (1978). Yogaville, Virginia: Internal Yoga Publications, p. 127.

9 Ibid, p. 128.

10 *Katha Upanishad*, 3.3–4. Translated by Patrick Olivelle in *Upanishads*, 1996. Oxford: Oxford University Press, pp. 238–40.

11 Komjathy, op cit.

12 The concept of a mandala representing the self was introduced by Carl Jung, who often used mandalas in his work and was influenced by Daoist theories of the self and the universe. Mandalas were motifs whose squared circles reflected the totality of an individual and an archetype of wholeness. Psychologist Kwang-Kuo Hwang broadened Jung's ideas and created a mandala for exploring the relationship of individual psychology and cultural context. See Jung, C., 1972. *Mandala Symbolism*,USA: Bollingen Foundation, Princeton University Press; Coward, H., 'Taoism and Jung: Synchronicity and the Self', *Philosophy East and West*, Vol. 46, No. 4, 1996, pp. 477–95. JSTOR, www.jstor.org/stable/1399493; Storr, A., 1983. *The Essential Jung*, 1998 (1983), London: Fontana Press, pp. 327–8; and Hwang, K., 'The Mandala Model of Self', in *Psychological Studies* (2011) 56: 329. Available at https://doi.org/10.1007/s12646-011-0110-1 [Accessed 9 July 2018].

13 Salzberg, S., *Lovingkindness: The Revolutionary Art of Happiness*, 2002. Boulder: Shambhala Publications, p. 23.

14 *Sutta Nipata (Karaniya Mettā Sutta)*, 1 Translated by Thanissaro Bhikkhu. Access to Insight. Available at https://www.accessto insight.org/tipitaka/kn/snp/snp.1.08.than.html.

15 In Ivanhoe, P. J., 6A8, *Confucian Moral Self Cultivation*, 2000. Hackett Publishing Company, Inc., [Kindle edition] p. 20.

16 Krishnamurti, J., *The Awakening of Intelligence*, 2011. [Ebook] p. 51. Available at https://www.scribd.com/read/385370079/Awakening-of-Intelligence#

17 Hanh, T. N., *Peace is Every Step: The Path of Mindfulness in Everyday Life*, 1991. United States and Canada: Bantam Books, pp. 73–7.

18 In Ivanhoe, P. J., op cit, 2A2: p. 21.

19 Kwo, D. W., *Chinese Brushwork in Painting and Calligraphy: Its History, Aesthetics and Techniques*, 1981. New York: Dover Publications, p. 249.

20 'Embodied Cognition' on the Liberated Body Podcast, Episode 59. Available at https://www.liberatedbody.com/podcast/cathy-kerr-lbp-056. Also, see Merchant, J., 'Mindfulness and meditation dampen down inflammation genes', *New Scientist*, 16 June 2017. Available at https://www.newscientist.com/article/2137595-mindfulness-and-meditation-dampen-down-inflammation-genes/ [Accessed 21 August 2018].

21 Farhi, D., *Bringing Yoga to Life: The Everyday Practice of Enlightened Living*, 2003. San Francisco: HarperSanFrancisco, p. 48.

Part 2: Xiu Yang for a Healthy and Harmonious Body

22 See Zheng Xuan's commentary to the *Liji* (*Book of Rites*), in Ishida, H., 'Body and Mind: The Chinese Perspective', in *Taoist Meditation and Longevity Techniques*, edited by Livia Kohn, 1989. Ann Arbour: Center for Chinese Studies, The University of Michigan, p. 45.

23 Keown, D., *The Spark in the Machine: How the Science of Acupuncture Explains the Mysteries of Western Medicine*, 2014. London: Singing Dragon, pp. 31, 78.

24 Lorenzo, M. et al., 'Osteoimmunology: Interactions of the Bone and Immune System', June 2008. National Institute of Health [online]. Available at https://www.ncbi.nlm.nih.gov/pmc/articles/ PMC2528852/ [Accessed 29 September 2018].

25 Mallinson, J. and Singleton, M., *Roots of Yoga*, 2017. UK: Penguin Random House, p. 127.

26 For more on bone-strengthening practices see Krucoff, C., 'Stand Strong: Yoga for Bone Health – Keep young and aging bones healthy with these yoga poses', 24 July 2013. *Yoga Journal* [online]. Available at https://www.Yogajournal.com/poses/standing-strong [Accessed 6 September 2018].

27 See Zhao E., Xu H., Wang L. et al., 'Bone marrow and the control of immunity', in *Cellular and Molecular Immunology*, January 2012, 9(1), 11–19. Available at https://www.ncbi.nlm.nih.gov/pmc/ articles/PMC3251706/ [Accessed 7 September 2018].

28 'Alcohol and Crime: Data from 2002 to 2008'. Available at https:// www.bjs.gov/content/acf/18_time_of_day.cfm [Accessed 4 January 2019]; National Press Release, 'Inaugural Compilation of Annual Crime Statistics from the National Incident-based Reporting System', 19 August 2013. Available at https:// archives.fbi.gov/archives/news/pressrel/press-releases/ fbi-releases-inaugural-compilation-of-annual-crime-statistics-from-the-national-incident-based-reporting-system [Accessed 4 January 2019].

29 *Nei-yeh (Inward Training)*, III.5, in *Original Tao: Inward Training and the Foundations of Taoist Mysticism*, 1999. Translated by Harold D. Roth. New York: Colombia University Press, p. 50.

30 Komjathy, op cit, Chapter 17.

31 Lewis, D., *The Tao of Natural Breathing: For Health, Well-Being and Inner Growth*, 2016. Boulder: Shambhala Publications, [Kindle for Mac]. p. 31. Retrieved from Amazon.co.uk.

32 Ibid, p. 42.

33 Farhi, D., *The Breathing Book*: *Good Health and Vitality Through Essential Breath Work*, 1996. New York: Henry Holt and Company, pp. 45–6.

34 Lewis, D., op cit, p. 42.

35 *Inward Training (Neiye)*, op cit, XX1.10–12, p. 86.

36 Translation by Maoshing Ni in *The Yellow Emperor's Classic of Medicine: A New Translation of the Neijing Suwen with Commentary*, 1995. Boulder: Shambhala Publications, Chapter 1, p. 2.

37 'Longevity Techniques in Japan', in Kohn, L., op cit, Chapter 1, p. 17. Translated by Sakade.

38 'How Greece Shaped Our Idea of the Body Beautiful', 5 June 2015. BBC.com. Available at http://www.bbc.com/culture/story/20150605-is-this-the-ideal-body [Accessed 5 September 2018].

39 Cohen, K., *The Way of Qigong: The Art and Science of Chinese Energy Healing*, 1997. New York: Balantine Books, p. 199.

40 Buric, I., Farias, M. et al., 'What Is the Molecular Signature of Mind–Body Interventions? A Systematic Review of Gene Expression Changes Induced by Meditation and Related Practices', in *Frontiers in Immunology*, 16 June 2017 [online]. Available at https://www.frontiersin.org/articles/10.3389/fimmu.2017.00670/full#B42 [Accessed 14 September 2018].

41 See https://journals.plos.org/plosone/article?id=10.1371/journal.pone.0120655 and https://www.nytimes.com/2018/09/10/well/move/using-tai-chi-to-build-strength.html [Both accessed 14 September 2018].

42 Wong, C., Schmid, C. H. et al., 'Comparative Effectiveness of Tai Chi Versus Physical Therapy for Knee Osteoarthritis: A Randomized Trial', in *Annals of Internal Medicine*, 19 July 2016. Available at https://annals.org/aim/article-abstract/2522435/comparative-effectiveness-tai-chi-versus-physical-therapy-knee-osteoarthritis-randomized [Accessed 14 September 2018].

43 See Wojtek, J. et al., 'Exercise and Physical Activity for Older Adults', American College of Sports Medicine, Position Stand, 2009. [PDF] Available at https://www.bewegenismedicijn.nl/files/downloads/acsm_position_stand_exercise_and_physical_activity_for_older_adults.pdf [Accessed 14 September 2018].

44 Despeux, C., 'Gymnastics: The Ancient Tradition', in *Taoist Meditation and Longevity Techniques*, op cit, p. 226.

45 Zhuangzi 11, 390, in Weingarten, O., '"Self-cultivation" (*Xiu Shen* 修身) in the Early Edited Literature: Uses and Contexts', in *Oriens Extremus* 54, 2015, p. 196. Available at http://oriens-extremus.org/wp-content/uploads/2017/11/OE-54-7.pdf. [Accessed 9 July 2018].

46 Kohn, L., *Chinese Healing Exercises*, 2008. Honolulu: University of Hawai'i Press, pp. 11–12.

47 Despeux, 22.1512, op cit, p. 239.

48 Ni, M., op cit, Chapter 22, p. 94.

49 Zhao, M., *Chinese Diet Therapy*, 1996. Beijing: China Esperanto Press. Translated by Jingen Wen.

50 Komjathy, op cit, p. 43.

51 Kastner, J., *Chinese Nutrition Therapy*, second edition, 2009. Stuttgart, Germany: Georg Thieme Verlag, p. 39.

52 American Dental Association, 'Saliva', MouthHealthy. Available at https://www.mouthhealthy.org/en/az-topics/s/saliva [Accessed 17 September 2018].

53 Zelman, K., 'Slow Down, You Eat Too Fast', WebMD. Available at https://www.webmd.com/diet/obesity/features/slow-down-you-eat-too-fast#1 [Accessed 24 September 2018].

54 Pedersen, A. M., Bardow, A. et al., 'Salivary and gastrointestinal functions of taste, mastication, swallowing and digestion', in *Oral Diseases*, 2002, 8 (3), 117–29. [PDF] Available at https://onlinelibrary.wiley.com/doi/epdf/10.1034/j.1601-0825.2002.02851.x [Accessed 24 September 2018].

55 Hanh, T. N., op cit, p. 24.

56 *Huang Ti Nei Ching Su Wen: The Yellow Emperor's Classic of Internal Medicine*, 1975, Book 7, Chapter 23. Translated by Ilza Veith. Oakland, California: University of California Press, p. 207.

57 Ibid.

58 Kastner, J., op cit, pp. 22–4.

59 Ni, M., op cit, Chapter 4, pp. 15–16.

60 Ibid.

Part 3: Xiu Yang for a Balanced Mental and Emotional Life

61 Schiffmann, E., *Yoga: The Spirit and Practice of Moving Into Stillness*, 1996. New York: Pocket Books, pp. 9–10.

62 1.2, *Yogaś citta vṛitti nirodaḥ*: 'Yoga is the restriction of the fluctuations of consciousness'. Translated by Georg Feuerstein in Feuerstein, G., *The Yoga Tradition: Its History, Literature, Philosophy and Practice*, 2001 (1998). Prescott, Arizona: Hohm Press, p. 217.

63 Kirov, B., *Heraclitus: Quotes and Facts*, 2016.: [Ebook] p. 20. Available on Scribd at https://www.scribd.com/read/339840142/ Heraclitus-Quotes-Facts#t_search-menu_420908n [Accessed 20 September 2018].

64 Translated by Bhikkhu, T. Available at https://www.dhammatalks. org/suttas/MN/MN118.html

65 Goldstein, J., *Mindfulness: A Practical Guide to Awakening*, 2013. Boulder, Colorado: Sounds True, p. 50.

66 Based on instructions in the *Satipaṭṭāna Sutta (M I 55–63).* Translated by Rupert Gethin in *Sayings of the Buddha: New translations from the Pali Nikāyas,* 2008. Oxford: Oxford University Press, p. 143.

67 Komjathy, op cit, p. 34.

68 Kornfield, J., *The Wise Heart*, 2008. [Kindle edition] p. 382. Retrieved from Amazon.co.uk.

69 See Kerr, C. et al., 'Mindfulness Starts with the Body: Somatosensory Attention and Top-down Modulation of Cortical Alpha Rhythms in Mindfulness Meditation', in *Frontiers in Human Neuroscience*, 13 February 2013, where she cites many of the clinical trials and studies that support this. Available at https:// www.frontiersin.org/articles/10.3389/fnhum.2013.00012/full. Also see McGreevey, S., 'Eight Weeks to a Better Brain' in Harvard Gazette, 21 Jan 2011. Available at https://news.harvard. edu/gazette/story/2011/01/eight-weeks-to-a-better-brain/ [Accessed 31 Jan 2019].

70 See Lieberman, M. et al., 'Putting Feelings Into Words: Affect Labeling Disrupts Amygdala Activity in Respose to Affective Stimuli', in *Psychological Science*, 2007, University of California, Los Angeles. Available at http://www.scn.ucla.edu/pdf/ AL%282007%29.pdf [Accessed 30 September 2018].

71 Liberated Body Podcast, op cit.

72 See Varela, F., Thompson, E. et al., *The Embodied Mind: Cognitive Science and Human Experience*, 2017. Cambridge and London: The MIT Press.

73 Komjathy, op cit, Chapter 3, p. 32.

74 https://en.oxforddictionaries.com/definition/emotion.

75 Komjathay, op. cit. p.33.

76 Chillot, R., 'The Power of Touch', in *Psychology Today*, 1 March 2013 (reviewed 5 October 2015). Available at https://www. psychologytoday.com/intl/articles/201303/the-power-touch [Accessed 26 September 2018].

77 *CBS News*, 'The Connection Between Busy Hands and Brain Chemistry', 19 August 2018. Available at https://www.cbsnews.com/news/the-connection-between-busy-hands-and-brain-chemistry/.

78 Eliot, T. S., *Four Quartets: Burnt Norton*, IV. [Kindle edition] Retrieved from Amazon.co.uk.

79 Coleman, M., *Make Peace with Your Mind*, 2016. Navato, California: New World Library, p. 20.

80 Marano, H. E., 'Our Brain's Negative Bias', in *Psychology Today*, 20 June 2003. Available at https://www.psychologytoday.com/us/articles/200306/our-brains-negative-bias [Accessed 27 September 2018].

Part 4: Xiu Yang for a Happier Place in the World

81 Dalai Lama and Cutler H. C., *The Art of Happiness*,1998. New York: Riverhead Books, p. 13.

82 Dass, R., *Polishing the Mirror*, 2013. Sounds True, [Kindle edition] p. 55.

83 Whyte, D., 'Sweet Darkness', in *The House of Belonging*, 2011. Langley, Washington: Many Rivers Press, p. 23.

84 See Hwang, K., 'Self-Cultivation: Culturally Sensitive Psychotherapies in Confucian Societies', in *The Counseling Psychologist*, 2009, Vol. 37, No. 7. Available at http://journals.sagepub.com/doi/abs/10.1177/0011000009339976 [Accessed 9 July 2018].

85 See Confucius, *The Analects*, 12.22. Translated with an introduction by D. C. Lau., 1979. London: Penguin Books, pp. 116–17.

86 Ibid, 2.1, p. 63.

87 *Zhongyu 20*, in Weingarten, O., op cit, p. 169.

88 Komjathy, op. cit, p. 35.

89 Salzberg, S., op cit, p. 156.

90 See Ishida, H., op cit, pp. 41–71.

91 Translated by Stephen Mitchell, *Tao Te Ching: A New English Version*, 2006. New York: Harper Perennial Modern Classics, Chapter 78.

92 See Csikszentmihalyi, M., *Flow: The Classic Work on How to Achieve Happiness*, 2002. USA: Harper & Row.

93 Lau, op cit, XXIX: 68, XXII: 50b, pp. 79, 87.

94 *Abhyasa* is practice, and *vairaghyam* is letting go. See *The Yoga Sutrā of Patanjali*, op cit, I.12–I.16.

95 Mitchell, S., op cit, Chapter 9.

96 Ibid.

97 Oliver, M., *New and Selected Poems, Volume One*, 1992. Boston, Massachusetts: Beacon Press, p. 68.

98 Hammer, M., 'The Enhancement of Spontaneity and Creativity', in *Journal of Psychology and Clinical Psychiatry*, Vol. 3, Issue 5, 2015, [PDF], p. 1. Available at https://medcraveonline.com/JPCPY/ JPCPY-03-00168.php [Accessed 16 October 2018].

99 Zhuangzi, *Inner Chapters*, in Wong, E., *Being Taoist: Wisdom for Living a Balanced Life*, 2015. Boston, Massachusetts: Shambhala Publications, p. 122.

100 *Samyutta Nikaya* 45.5, *Anguttara Nikaya* 5.198. Translated by Bhikku, B.

101 From 'Nourishing Life', in Wong, E., op cit, p. 126.

102 Komjathy, op cit, Chapter 9, p. 35..

103 Suzuki, S. *Zen Mind, Beginner's Mind*, 2006. Boston: Shambhala Publications, p. 21.

104 Sagmeister, S., 'The Power of Time Off', TED.com. Available at https://www.ted.com/talks/stefan_sagmeister_the_power_of_ time_off [Accessed 29 May 2018].

105 *The Enlightened Mind: An Anthology of Sacred Prose*, edited by Stephen Mitchell, 1991. New York: HarperCollins Publishers, p. 98.

106 Krishnamurti, J., *Total Freedom*, 1996. Ojai, California: Krishnamurti Foundation of America, p. 288.

107 Huxley, A., *The Doors of Perception: Heaven and Hell,* 1954. Vintage Classics, [Kindle edition], p. 8.

108 Hemenway, T., *Gaia's Garden: A Guide to Homescale Permaculture*, second edition, 2009 (2000). White River Junction, Vermont: Chelsea Green Publishing, pp. 184–5.

109 Little, B., *Companion Planting*, 2008. London: Hew Holland Publishers (UK) Ltd, p. 27.

110 Kornfield, J., 'Finding Freedom, Love, and Joy in the Present Moment', Tim Ferriss Show Podcast. Transcript of show available at https://tim.blog/2018/06/04/the-tim-ferriss-show-transcripts- jack-kornfield/ [Accessed 31 December 2018].

111 Mitchell, S., op cit, Chapter 11.

112 Hanh, T. N., *The Heart of the Buddha's Teachings: Transforming Suffering into Peace, Joy & Liberation: The Four Noble Truths, The Noble Eightfold Path, and Other Basic Buddhist Teachings*, 1998. New York: Broadway Books, p. 136.

Conclusion: From Inner Balance to Outer Radiance

113 Komjathy, op cit, Chapter 12.

FURTHER READING

Cohen, K., 1997. *The Way of Qigong: The Art and Science of Chinese Energy Healing.* New York: Ballantine Books.

Coleman, M., 2016. *Make Peace with Your Mind: How Mindfulness and Compassion Can Free You from Your Inner Critic.* Navato, California: New World Library.

Farhi, D., 1996. *The Breathing Book: Good Health and Vitality Through Essential Breath Work.* New York: Henry Holt and Company.

Farhi, D., 2001. *Yoga Mind, Body and Spirit: A Return to Wholeness.* New York: Henry Holt and Company.

Farhi, D., 2003. *Bringing Yoga to Life: The Everyday Practice of Enlightened Living.* San Francisco: HarperSanFrancisco.

Goldsmith, E. and Klein, M., 2017. *Nutritional Healing with Chinese Medicine.* Ontario, Canada: Robert Rose Inc.

Goldstein, J., 2013. *Mindfulness: A Practical Guide to Awakening.* Boulder, Colorado: Sounds True.

Hanh, T. N., 1991. *Peace is Every Step: The Path of Mindfulness in Everyday Life.* United States and Canada: Bantam Books.

Hanh, T. N., 1999. *The Heart of the Buddha's Teachings.* New York: Broadway Books.

Hanh, T. N., 2008. *Breathe, You Are Alive! The Sutrā on the Full Awareness of Breathing.* Berkeley, California: Parallax Press.

Hwang, K., 2001. 'The Mandala Model of Self', in *Psychological Studies* (2011) 56: 329.

Inward Training (Neiye). Translation by Louis Komjathy, 2008 (2003). In *Handbooks for Daoist Practice*, Volume 1. Hong Kong: Yuen Yuen Institute.

Ivanhoe, P. J., 2000. *Confucian Moral Self Cultivation.* USA: Hackett Publishing Company, Inc.

Jung, C., 1972. *Mandala Symbolism*. USA: Bollingen Foundation, Princeton University Press.

Kastner, J., MD, LaC, 2009. *Chinese Nutritional Therapy: Dietetics in Traditional Chinese Medicine (TCM)*, second edition. Stuttgart, Germany: Georg Thieme Verlag.

Kirkland, R., 2003. *Taoism: The Enduring Tradition*. London: Routledge.

Kohn, L., 2008. *Chinese Healing Exercises: The Tradition of Daoyin*. Honolulu: University of Hawai'i Press.

Kuo-Deemer, M., 2018. *Qigong and the Tai Chi Axis: Nourishing Practices for Body, Mind and Spirit*. London: Orion Spring.

Lao Tzu Tao Te Ching, 1963. Translated by D. C. Lau. London: Penguin Books Ltd.

Reichstein, G., 1998. *Wood Becomes Water: Chinese Medicine in Everyday Life*. New York: Kodansha America, Inc.

Roth, H. D., 1991. 'Psychology and Self-Cultivation in Early Taoistic Thought', *Harvard Journal of Asiatic Studies* 51.

Roth, H. D., 1999. *Original Tao: Inward Training and the Foundations of Taoist Mysticism*. New York; Chichester: Columbia University Press.

Salzberg, S., 2002. *Lovingkindness: The Revolutionary Art of Happiness*. Boulder: Shambhala Publications.

Schiffmann, E., 1996. *Yoga: The Spirit and Practice of Moving Into Stillness*. New York: Pocket Books.

Tao Te Ching. Translation by Stephen Mitchell, 1998. New York: Harper Perennial Modern Classics.

Wong, E., 2015. *Being Taoist: Wisdom for Living a Balanced Life*. Boston, Massachusetts: Shambhala Publications.

ADDITIONAL RESOURCES

Daoism, Chinese medicine and qigong resources

Cohen, Kenneth. Qigong Healing website. www.qigonghealing.com
Cohen, Matthew. Sacred Energy Arts. www.sacredenergyarts.com
Kuo-Deemer, Mimi. *Qigong Basics* and *Qigong Flow* DVDs/
downloadable videos. Available on Vimeo and Amazon. Includes
the Eighteen Forms, Eight Brocades, Five Elements Qigong and
Five Elements Mudras.
Kuo-Deemer, Mimi. YouTube qigong videos. Available at
www.youtube.com/mimikuodeemer.

Yoga resources

Farhi, Donna. Video tutorials available at www.donnafarhi.co.nz/
product-category/videos
Kuo-Deemer, Mimi. MovementforModernLife.com – online qigong
and yoga videos.
Kuo-Deemer, Mimi. *Finding Balance: Yoga, Qigong and Mindfulness*
DVD/downloadable videos. Available on Vimeo and Amazon.
Schiffmann, Erich. www.erichschiffmann.com and
www.yogaanytime.com – online yoga videos and talks.

Mindfulness resources

Meditation apps
• Insight Timer
• Calm
• The Mindfulness App

Aylward, Martin. Online dharma talks. www.martinaylward.com/
    listen.
Worldwide Insight. Weekly online courses www.worldwideinsight.org
Dharma Seed. Western Buddhist Vipassana Teachings.
    www.dharmaseed.org

ACKNOWLEDGEMENTS

My brother Jay once asked my mother, who at the time was eighty-one years old, whether she believes in fate. With a sweet conviction and smile, she replied, 'Of course.' What she referred to as fate, however, is closer to what in Chinese is known as *yuan fen* (緣分) – a karmic turn or chance meeting that brings things or people together. *Yuan fen* is what I believe has made writing this book and the culmination of ideas in it possible.

Generationally, my *yuan fen* has blessed me with my family. My mother, who – among many things in her life – was a writer. She published hundreds of short stories and essays in the Chinese overseas press describing her life and observations of Chinese culture, society and its role and place in the world. I'd like to thank her for inspiring the gift of knowing the world through language and storytelling. I also want to thank her for giving me her photocopied yoga book from the 1970s. Her gift was indeed *yuan fen*, for that book started me on a path that would alter my life indescribably.

I also want to thank my father. As one of his friends once described, my father was a true Confucian gentleman – humble, kind, filial and deeply learned. To me, his qualities were the result of his own forms of xiu yang. Through him, I learned by example to listen and see beyond the surface of ideas. Though he was a scientist through and through, I also knew him to have a deep respect for nature and the principles underlying Daoism and Buddhism. If it were not for the many cross-country trips that involved hiking, camping in national parks and frequently stopping to admire and photograph tall, old trees, I may have never grown up appreciating what I do. I hope that wherever his spirit is today, I have and will continue to honour his life.

I am also fortunate to have my three older brothers, Jay, Kaiser and John. They have been a steady influence in my life, directing and focusing my interests and shaping the landscape of my ideas. As their only sister and youngest of the bunch, their humour, achievements and values are and have always been astonishing to me. I have enormous respect for the way they continually work towards positive change in the world.

It is also *yuan fen* that led me on the path of xiu yang. It started with doing yoga regularly in Los Angeles; for this, I have to thank one of my best friends for over thirty years, Melissa Donfeld Cherry. I also have to thank Robyn Wexler, another one of my closest friends in life. As it happened, it was during a meeting with a Green Peace representative in Berkeley, California, that we decided to open our yoga school in Beijing, Yoga Yard. That day's decision radically changed the trajectory of my practice and teaching in ways I would never have imagined possible.

I believe the fate and the workings of *yuan fen* also bring the teachers we admire and trust into our lives. I thank my academic professors at SOAS: Dr Ulrich Pagel, Dr Antonello Palumbo and Dr Theodore Proferes. I also thank my spiritual teachers – who include Erich Schiffmann, Donna Farhi, Matthew Cohen, Cameron Tukapua, Max Strom, Martin Aylward and Mark Coleman – for their wisdom, love and continual inspiration. I am especially grateful to Donna Farhi, who generously wrote the foreword for this book. Our *yuan fen* has blossomed into an exceptional gift. After one workshop with her and a dinner in California, we spawned a relationship that has spanned fifteen years and crossed four continents. I am immeasurably appreciative to Donna for inspiring the direction of my work, and for her continual encouragement to me to write.

Yuan fen also helped form the concept for *Xiu Yang*. It was during a lively meeting with my agent, Anna Hogarty, and soon-to-be-editor, Olivia Morris, about my first book, *Qigong and the Tai Chi Axis*, that the seeds for *Xiu Yang* were planted. I would like to extend my deep appreciation to both of them for the vision and faith to grow this book into being. I would also like to thank Amanda Harris, Ru Merritt and Alex Layt at Orion Spring for their dedication and support, Emanuel Santos for the exquisite illustrations in the book, and my Uncle Peter for the beautiful calligraphy.

Fate has also brought me the honour of knowing and working with many people for whom I am grateful. This includes the producers at New Shoot Pictures, Christine Romano and Matt Wright and Kat Farrants at Movement for Modern Life; their videos have brought more visibility to many of the xiu yang practices I have included in this book. It also includes many at triyoga in London, such as Jonathan Sattin and Genny Wilkinson-Priest, as well as those at The Life Centre such as Elizabeth Stanley and Graham Burns, and Jo Manuel at the Special Yoga Centre.

Through many avenues I have also had the blessing of treasured friendship with James Rafael, Jen Copestake and Charlotte Wu. James and Jen kindly read and redacted early versions of my manuscript, and Charlotte gently helped give the book's outline and themes a stronger backbone. I am indebted to them for their camaraderie, astuteness and all-around fabulousness.

To my friends I have not yet mentioned – thank you for indulging me with dumplings and other Chinese feasts, shared time on retreats and trainings, and – most of all – for your precious, precious love, support and laughter. Our stars have aligned in ways I am forever grateful for. I also wish to remember my dear friend Mayling Birney, who passed on from this life in 2017. I wish I could thank her in person for all she was to me and the many who loved her. Her clear intellect, piercing loyalty, radiant smile and continual investment in all things generous, joyful and kind are a continuous source of inspiration and goodness that I can only hope to grow and cultivate as beautifully as she did.

Lastly, my most treasured *yuan fen* has been having Aaron Deemer as my partner through life. There is also no one in the world who knows me better, and no one better suited to helping me stay true to who I am. For this, I thank him from the depths, heights and mysteries of the Dao.

ABOUT THE AUTHOR

Mimi Kuo-Deemer is dedicated to living, sharing and evolving the art of xiu yang. She champions the balance of playfulness and precision as the best way forward in life, and never underestimates how sitting, breathing and conscious movement can provide the clearest and most compassionate perspective on the messy, complex and often unpredictable job of being human. She is a teacher of both students and other teachers, having practised and taught yoga, qigong and meditation for over twenty years in China, the UK, Europe and the United States. In 1994, she graduated from Stanford University and, in 2016, she received an MA with distinction from SOAS in Traditions of Yoga and Meditation. Originally from Tucson, Arizona, she lived in China for over fourteen years where she worked as a photojournalist as well act as co-founding and co-directing Yoga Yard, Beijing's first and leading yoga studio. Mimi now lives in the UK, where she is a senior teacher at triyoga, London's pre-eminent centre for health and well-being, and a regular contributor to the online platform, Movement for Modern Life. *Xiu Yang: Self-cultivation for a happier, healthier and balanced life* is her second book.

Qigong and the Tai Chi Axis

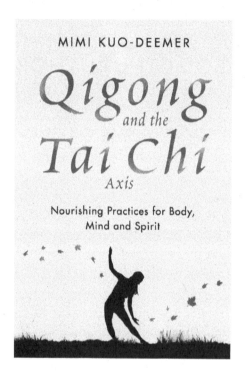

MIMI KUO-DEEMER

Qigong
and the
Tai Chi
Axis

Nourishing Practices for Body,
Mind and Spirit

**Reduce stress, release pain and create whole body
harmony with this practical introduction to Qigong and
the yin/yang balance of Tai Chi, the ancient Chinese
arts of 'movement meditation'.**

From reducing stress and improving posture to balance
and general mobility, the many physical and mental benefits
of Qigong and Tai Chi are widely celebrated. In this accessible
book, Mimi Kuo-Deemer offers practices, insights and wisdom
on these arts, and shows us how to support our natural
capacity for energy, balance and well-being.